A Pocket Guide to

PHYSICAL EXAMINATION AND HISTORY TAKING

A Pocket Guide to

PHYSICAL EXAMINATION AND HISTORY TAKING

Barbara Bates, M.D.

Lecturer in Medicine, Department of Medicine
University of Pennsylvania School of Medicine

Lecturer in Nursing
University of Pennsylvania School of Nursing
Philadelphia, Pennsylvania

WITH PEDIATRIC CONTENT BY

Robert A. Hoekelman, M.D.

Professor and Chairman, Department of Pediatrics
University of Rochester School of Medicine and Dentistry

Professor of Nursing
University of Rochester School of Nursing
Rochester, New York

J. B. LIPPINCOTT Philadelphia
New York • London • Hagerstown

Acquisitions Editor: Donna L. Hilton, R.N., B.S.N.
Coordinating Editorial Assistant: Barbara Nelson Cullen
Project Editor: Dina Kamilatos
Manuscript Editor: Mary Norris
Indexer: Katherine Pitcoff
Art Director: Ellen C. Dawson
Designer: Ellen C. Dawson and Kathy Kelley-Luedtke
Design Coordinator: Kathy Kelley-Luedtke
Production Manager: Caren Erlichman
Production Coordinator: Sharon McCarthy
Compositor: Tapsco, Incorporated
Printer/Binder: R. R. Donnelley & Sons Company

6   5   4   3

Library of Congress Cataloging-in-Publication Data

Bates, Barbara
  A pocket guide to physical examination and history taking /
Barbara Bates; with pediatric content by Robert A. Hoekelman.
    p.   cm.
  Includes bibliographical references and index.
  ISBN 0-397-54783-8
  1. Physical diagnosis—Handbooks, manuals, etc.
  2. Medical history taking—Handbooks, manuals, etc.
  I. Hoekelman, Robert A.   II.   Title.
  RC76.B38   1991
  616.07′54—dc20   90-6611
                                                              CIP

Any procedure or practice described in this book should be applied by the
health-care practitioner under appropriate supervision in accordance with
professional standards of care with regard to the unique circumstances that
apply in each practice situation. Care has been taken to confirm the
accuracy of information presented and to describe accepted practices.
However, the authors, editors, and publisher cannot accept any
responsibility for errors or omissions or for any consequences from
application of the information in this book and make no warranty, express
or implied, with respect to the contents of the book.

Every effort has been made to ensure drug selections and dosages are in
accordance with current recommendations and practice. Because of
ongoing research, changes in government regulations and the constant
flow of information on drug therapy, reactions and interactions, the reader
is cautioned to check the package insert for each drug for indications,
dosages, warnings and precautions, particularly if the drug is new or
infrequently used.

ACKNOWLEDGMENT

We appreciate the help of Barbara L. Brush, R.N.C., M.S.N., in selecting illustrations and reviewing some of the text.

CONTENTS

INTRODUCTION

The *Pocket Guide to Physical Examination and History Taking* is a concise, portable text that

- Outlines the health history
- Provides an illustrated review of the physical examination
- Reminds students of some common findings
- Describes some of the special techniques of assessment that the student may need in specific instances but may not recall in sufficient detail
- Provides succinct aids to interpretation of selected findings

There are several ways to use the *Pocket Guide*:

- To review and thus remember the content of a health history
- To review and rehearse the techniques of examination. This can be done while learning a single section and again while combining the approaches to several body systems or regions into an integrated examination.
- To review some common variations of normal and some selected abnormalities. Observation is more astute when the examiner knows what to look, listen, and feel for.

- To look up special maneuvers as the need arises. Techniques such as everting an eyelid or doing an Allen test are included in the relevant sections of the examination and are initiated by a gray bar. This bar helps readers to use or ignore the special maneuvers, as they prefer.
- To look up additional information about possible findings, including abnormalities and standards of normal

The *Pocket Guide* is not intended to serve as a primary text from which to learn the skills of taking a history or performing a physical examination. Its detail is insufficient for these purposes. It is intended instead as a mechanism for review and recall and as a convenient, brief, and portable reference.

1

The Health History

Taking a history is usually the first and often the most important part of your interaction with patients. You gather much of the data on which diagnoses are based, you learn about the patients as people and how they have experienced their symptoms and illnesses, and you begin to establish a trusting relationship.

There are several ways to facilitate these goals. Try to provide an environment that is private, quiet, and free of interruption. Seat yourself in a location that is agreeable to the patient, and make sure that he or she is comfortable. Address the patient by name and title, *e.g.*, Mrs. Green, and introduce yourself.

Start the history with open-ended questions: "What brings you to the hospital? . . . Anything else? . . . Tell me about it." Additional ways of encouraging patients to tell their stories include:

Facilitation—posture, actions, or words that communicate interest, such as leaning forward, making eye contact, or saying "Mm-hmmm" or "Go on"

Reflection—repetition of a word or phrase that a patient has used

Clarification—asking what the patient meant by a word or phrase

Empathic responses—recognizing through actions or words the feelings of a patient, such as by offering a tissue or saying "I understand" or "That must have been frightening"

Asking about feelings that a patient has had regarding symptoms, events, or other matters

Confrontation—identifying something about the patient's behavior or feelings not expressed verbally or apparently inconsistent with the patient's story

Interpretation—putting into words what you infer about the patient's feelings or about the meaning to the patient of symptoms, events, or other matters

To get specific details, direct questions are often necessary.

- Word them in language understandable to the patient.
- Express them neutrally so as not to lead the patient.
- Ask about one item at a time.
- Proceed from the general to the specific.
- Ask for graded responses rather than a simple "Yes" or "No." Multiple-choice questions may also be used.

———— *A Comprehensive History of an Adult* ————

DATE of the history

IDENTIFYING DATA: age, sex, race, place of birth, marital status, occupation, and religion

SOURCE OF REFERRAL, if any

SOURCE of the history

RELIABILITY of the history

CHIEF COMPLAINT(S)

PRESENT ILLNESS: a clear, chronological narrative that includes the onset of the problem, the setting in which it developed, its manifestations, and any treatments. The principal symptoms should be described in terms of:

- Location
- Quality
- Quantity or severity
- Timing (onset, duration, frequency)
- Setting
- Factors that aggravated or relieved
- Associated manifestations

The present illness should also include the patient's under-standing of the symptoms and incapacities, his or her re-sponses to them, and the meaning and impact that they have had in the patient's life.

PAST HISTORY

General State of Health
Childhood Illnesses
Adult Illnesses
Psychiatric Illnesses
Accidents and Injuries
Operations
Hospitalizations

CURRENT HEALTH STATUS

Allergies
Immunizations, such as tetanus, pertussis, diphtheria, polio, measles, rubella, mumps, influenza, hepatitis B, *Hemophilus influenzae,* and pneumococcal vaccine

Screening Tests, such as hematocrit, urinalysis, tuberculin test, Pap smear, mammogram, cholesterol test, and test of stool for occult blood, with dates and results

Environmental Hazards in the home, school, and work-place

Use of Safety Measures, such as seat belts

Exercise and Leisure Activities

Sleep Patterns

Diet, including beverages, over a recent 24-hour period

Current Medications: home remedies, nonprescription drugs, vitamin and mineral supplements, prescribed drugs; use over a 24-hour period

Tobacco, including the type, amount, and duration of use

Alcohol and Illicit Drugs, including the type, amount, frequency, and duration of use

FAMILY HISTORY

- Age and health, or age and cause of death, of parents, siblings, spouse, and children. Data on other relatives may also be useful.
- The occurrence of diabetes, tuberculosis, heart disease, high blood pressure, stroke, kidney disease, cancer, arthritis, anemia, headaches, epilepsy, mental illness, alcoholism, drug addiction, and symptoms like those of the patient

PSYCHOSOCIAL HISTORY

Home Situation and Significant Others, including family and friends

Daily Life over a 24-hour period

Important Experiences, including upbringing, school, military service, work, financial situation, marriage, retirement

Religious Beliefs, if relevant

Outlook on the present and the future

REVIEW OF SYSTEMS

General. Usual weight, recent weight change, fatigue, fever

Skin. Rashes, lumps, sores, itching, dryness, color change, changes in hair or nails

Head. Headaches, head injury

Eyes. Vision, glasses or contact lenses, last eye examination, pain, redness, excessive tearing, double vision, glaucoma, cataracts

Ears. Hearing, tinnitus, vertigo, earaches, infection, discharge

Nose and Sinuses. Frequent colds; nasal stuffiness, discharge, itching; hay fever, nosebleeds, sinus trouble

Mouth and Throat. Condition of teeth and gums, bleeding gums, last dental examination, sore tongue, frequent sore throats, hoarseness

Neck. Lumps in the neck, "swollen glands," goiter, pain or stiffness in the neck

Breasts. Lumps, pain or discomfort, nipple discharge, self-examination

Respiratory. Cough, sputum (color, quantity), hemoptysis, wheezing, asthma, bronchitis, emphysema, pneumonia, tuberculosis, pleurisy; last chest x-ray

Cardiac. Heart trouble, high blood pressure, rheumatic fever, heart murmurs; chest pain or discomfort, palpitations; dyspnea, orthopnea, paroxysmal nocturnal dyspnea, edema; past ECG or other heart tests

Gastrointestinal. Trouble swallowing, heartburn, appetite, nausea, vomiting, regurgitation, vomiting of blood, indigestion. Frequency of bowel movements, color and size of stools, change in bowel habits, rectal bleeding or black tarry stools, hemorrhoids, constipation, diarrhea. Abdominal pain, food intolerance, excessive belching or passing of gas. Jaundice, liver or gallbladder trouble, hepatitis

Urinary. Frequency of urination, polyuria, nocturia, burning or pain on urination, hematuria, urgency, reduced caliber or force of the urinary stream, hesitancy, incontinence; urinary infections, stones

Genital, Male
- Hernias, penile discharge or sores, testicular pain or masses, any sexually transmitted diseases and their treatments, exposure to AIDS and precautions taken against it
- Sexual interest, orientation, function, satisfaction, and problems; contraceptive methods

Genital, Female

- Age at menarche; regularity, frequency, and duration of periods; amount of bleeding, bleeding between periods or after intercourse, last menstrual period; dysmenorrhea, premenstrual tension; age at menopause, menopausal symptoms, postmenopausal bleeding
- Discharge, itching, sores, lumps, any sexually transmitted diseases and their treatments, exposure to AIDS and precautions against it
- Number of pregnancies, number of deliveries, number of abortions (spontaneous and induced); complications of pregnancy; contraceptive methods
- Sexual interest, orientation, function, satisfaction; any problems, including dyspareunia

Peripheral Vascular. Intermittent claudication, leg cramps, varicose veins, clots in the veins

Musculoskeletal. Muscle or joint pains, stiffness, arthritis, gout, backache. If present, describe the location and symptoms (swelling, redness, pain, tenderness, stiffness, weakness, limitation of motion or activity).

Neurologic. Fainting, blackouts, seizures, weakness, paralysis, numbness, tingling, tremors or other involuntary movements

Hematologic. Anemia, easy bruising or bleeding, past transfusions and possible reactions

Endocrine. Thyroid trouble, heat or cold intolerance, excessive sweating; diabetes, excessive thirst or hunger, polyuria

Psychiatric. Nervousness, tension, mood including depression; memory

——— *A Comprehensive Pediatric History* ———

The child's history follows the same outline as the adult's history, with certain *additions* presented here.

IDENTIFYING DATA: Date and place of birth; nickname; first names of parents (and last name of each, if different)

CHIEF COMPLAINTS. Determine if they are the concerns of the child, the parent(s), a schoolteacher, or some other person.

PRESENT ILLNESS. Determine how each member of the family responds to the child's symptoms, why he or she is concerned, and the secondary gain the child may get from the illness.

PAST HISTORY

Birth History, important when neurologic or developmental problems are present. Get hospital records if necessary.

- Prenatal—maternal health, medications, drug and alcohol use, vaginal bleeding, weight gain
- Natal—nature of labor and delivery, birth weight
- Neonatal—resuscitation efforts, cyanosis, jaundice, infections; nature of bonding

Feeding History, important with under- and overnutrition

- Breast feeding—frequency and duration of feeds, difficulties encountered; timing and method of weaning
- Artificial feeding—type, amount, frequency; vomiting, colic, diarrhea; vitamin, iron, and fluoride supplements; introduction of solid foods
- Eating habits—likes and dislikes, types and amounts of food eaten; parental attitudes and response to feeding problems

Growth and Development History, important with delayed growth, psychomotor and intellectual retardation, and behavioral disturbances

- Physical growth—weight and height at birth and 1, 2, 5, and 10 years, periods of slow or rapid growth
- Developmental milestones—ages child held head up, rolled over, sat, stood, walked, and talked

- Social development—day and night sleeping patterns; toilet training; speech problems; habitual behaviors, discipline problems; school performance; relationships with parents, siblings, and peers

CURRENT HEALTH STATUS

Allergies. Pay particular attention to childhood allergies—eczema, urticaria, perennial allergic rhinitis, and insect hypersensitivity.

Immunizations. Include dates given and any untoward reactions.

Screening Tests. Include those for inborn errors of metabolism, sickle cell disease, blood lead, vision, and hearing.

2

The Physical Examination of an Adult

─────── *Overview* ───────

For a comprehensive physical examination, use a sequence that maximizes your efficiency and minimizes the patient's effort, yet allows you to be thorough. One such sequence is outlined below, together with symbols that indicate the patient's positions.

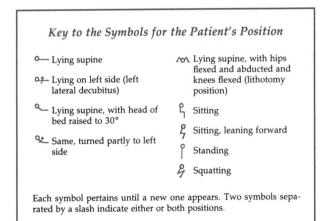

Key to the Symbols for the Patient's Position

○— Lying supine

○⌐ Lying on left side (left lateral decubitus)

◕— Lying supine, with head of bed raised to 30°

◕⌐ Same, turned partly to left side

〰 Lying supine, with hips flexed and abducted and knees flexed (lithotomy position)

Ꝑ Sitting

Ꝑ Sitting, leaning forward

ꝑ Standing

Ᵽ Squatting

Each symbol pertains until a new one appears. Two symbols separated by a slash indicate either or both positions.

For the first three sections of this examination, no specific position is necessary.

Sequence of a Comprehensive Examination

Mental Status

General Survey

Skin

� Head and Neck, including an initial survey of respirations

Musculoskeletal Examination of the neck, upper back, and possibly upper extremities; costovertebral angle tenderness

Posterior Thorax and Lungs

Breast Inspection, Axillae, and Epitrochlear Nodes

o— Breast Palpation

Anterior Thorax and Lungs

ᨆ Cardiovascular System

ᨆ • For finding an elusive apical impulse and for hearing a left-sided S_3 or S_4 and the murmur of mitral stenosis

ᨖ • For hearing the murmur of aortic regurgitation

o— Abdomen

o⨍ Male: Rectum

∧∧ Female: Genitalia and Rectum

o— Legs and Feet: peripheral vascular and musculoskeletal examination, and inspection for neurologic findings

ᨆ Spine, Legs, and Feet

Varicose Veins

Male: Genitalia and Hernias

Neurologic Screening, including gait and legs, Romberg test, and shoulders, arms, and hands

o—/ ᠙ Motor System

Reflexes

Sensory System

The rest of this chapter is devoted to the examination, unit by unit. To facilitate the review or rehearsal of individual body systems or regions, each is described as a whole. The Thorax and Lungs, for example, make up one unit. In practice, however, as shown in the overview above, examination of the breasts and axillae is interposed between the examinations of the posterior thorax and the anterior thorax. Such interpositions or other changes in order are indicated by colored shading in the following text.

———— *Mental Status* ————

—*Examination Techniques*—   —*Possible Findings*—

Observe patient's mental status during interview. Testing of specific functions may also follow interview or physical examination.

APPEARANCE AND BEHAVIOR

Assess the following:

Level of Consciousness. **Observe** patient's alertness and response to verbal stimuli. If necessary, touch or gently shake patient's arm or shoulder, or cause pain.

Normal consciousness, drowsiness (obtundation), stupor, coma

Posture and Motor Behavior. **Observe** pace, range, char-

Restlessness, agitation, bizarre postures, immobility,

·

—Examination Techniques—	—Possible Findings—
acter, and appropriateness of movements.	involuntary movements
Dress, Grooming, and Personal Hygiene	Fastidiousness, neglect
Facial Expression during rest and interaction	Anxiety, depression, elation, anger, responses to imaginary people or objects, withdrawal
Manner, Affect, and Relation to Persons and Things	

SPEECH AND LANGUAGE

Note quantity, rate, loudness, and fluency of speech. If indicated, test for aphasia.	Aphasia, dysphonia, dysarthria, changes with mood disorders

MOOD

Inquire about patient's spirits. *Note* nature, intensity, duration, and stability of any abnormal mood. If indicated, **assess** risk of suicide.	Happiness, elation, depression, anxiety, anger, indifference

THOUGHT AND PERCEPTIONS

Thought Processes. **Assess** logic, relevance, organization, and coherence of patient's thought.	Loosening of associations, flight of ideas, incoherence, confabulation, blocking
Thought Content. **Explore** or inquire about any unusual or unpleasant thoughts.	Obsessions, compulsions, delusions, feelings of unreality
Perceptions. **Inquire** about any unusual perceptions,	Illusions, hallucinations

—Examination Techniques—	—Possible Findings—

e.g., seeing or hearing things.

Insight and Judgment. **Assess** patient's insight into the illness and the level of judgment used in making decisions or plans.

Recognition or denial of the mental cause of symptoms; bizarre, impulsive, or unrealistic judgment

MEMORY AND ATTENTION

As indicated, **assess:**

Orientation to time, place, and person

Disorientation

Attention

- *Digit span*—the ability to repeat a series of numbers forward and then backward

- *Serial 7s*—the ability to subtract 7 repeatedly, starting with 100

- *Spelling backward* of a five-letter word, such as W-O-R-L-D

Poor performance of digit span, serial 7s, and spelling backward is common in dementia and delirium but has other causes too.

Remote Memory, e.g., birthdays, anniversaries, social security number, schools, jobs, wars

Impaired in late stages of dementia

Recent memory, e.g., events of the day

New learning ability—the ability to repeat three or

Recent memory and new learning ability are impaired in dementia and delirium, but impairment has other causes too.

—*Examination Techniques*—	—*Possible Findings*—

four words after a few minutes of unrelated activity

HIGHER COGNITIVE FUNCTIONS

As indicated, **assess:**

Information and Vocabulary. Note range and depth of patient's information, com- plexity of ideas expressed, and vocabulary used. For the fund of information you may also ask names of presidents, other political figures, or large cities.	These attributes reflect in- telligence, education, and cultural background. They are limited by mental retar- dation, but fairly well pre- served in early dementia.
Calculating Abilities, such as addition, subtraction, and multiplication	Poor calculations in mental retardation and dementia
Abstract Thinking—the abil- ity to respond abstractly to questions about	Concrete responses are common in mental retarda- tion, dementia, and delir- ium.

- The meaning of *proverbs,* such as "A stitch in time saves nine"

- The *similarities* of beings or things, such as a cat and a mouse or a piano and a violin

Constructional Ability. Ask patient	Impaired ability is common in dementia and with pari- etal lobe damage.

- To copy figures such as a circle, cross, diamond, box, and two intersecting pentagons, or

—Examination Techniques—   *—Possible Findings—*

- To draw a clock face with
  numbers and hands

———— *The General Survey* ————

Take **note** of the following
attributes during the interview and the physical ex-
amination. Pulse, blood
pressure, and respiratory
rate may be checked ini-
tially or later in the examination.

Apparent State of Health	Robust, acutely or chroni-cally ill, frail
Signs of Distress	Labored breathing, winc-ing, sweatiness, trembling
Skin Color	Pallor, cyanosis, jaundice
Stature and Habitus	Tall, short, muscular; dis-proportionately long limbs
Sexual Development	Facial hair, voice changes, breast development
Weight, by appearance or measurement	Emaciated, slender, plump, fat
Posture, Motor Activity, and Gait	Postures to ease breathing or pain, ataxia, a limp, pa-ralysis
Dress, Grooming, and Per-sonal Hygiene	Excessive clothes of hypo-thyroidism, long sleeves to cover a rash or needle marks
Odors of Body or Breath	Alcohol, odors of diabetic acidosis, uremia, liver fail-ure

—*Examination Techniques*—	—*Possible Findings*—
Facial Expression	Stare of hyperthyroidism, immobile face of parkinsonism
Speech	Fast speech of hyperthyroidism, hoarseness of myxedema

Vital Signs, including

• Pulse rate and blood pressure	Tachycardia, hypertension
• Respiratory rate	Tachypnea
• Temperature	Fever, hypothermia

——————— *The Skin* ———————

Examine each region.

SKIN

Inspect and **palpate. Note**

• Color	Cyanosis, changes in melanin
• Moisture	Moist, dry, oily
• Temperature	Cool, warm
• Texture	Smooth, rough
• Mobility—the ease with which a fold of skin can be moved	Decreased in edema
• Turgor—the speed with which the fold returns into place	Decreased in dehydration

Note any lesions, including

—*Examination Techniques*—	—*Possible Findings*—
• Anatomic location	Generalized, localized
• Grouping or arrangement	Linear, clustered, dermatomal
• Type	Macule, papule, bulla, tumor
• Color	Red, white, brown, mauve

NAILS

Inspect and **palpate** the fingernails and toenails. **Note**

• Color	Cyanosis, pallor
• Shape	Clubbing, spoon nails
• Any lesions	Splinter hemorrhages

HAIR

Inspect and **palpate** the hair. **Note**

• Quantity	Thin, thick
• Distribution	Patchy or total alopecia
• Texture	Fine, coarse

——— *The Head and Eyes* ———

♀ *HEAD*

Examine the

• Hair, including quantity, distribution, and texture	Coarse and sparse in myxedema, fine in hyperthyroidism

—Examination Techniques—	*—Possible Findings—*
• Scalp, including lumps or lesions	Sebaceous cysts, psoriasis
• Skull, including size and contour	Hydrocephalus, Paget's disease of bone
• Face, including symmetry and facial expression	Facial paralysis, emotions
• Skin, including color, texture, hair distribution, and lesions	Pale, fine, hirsute Acne, skin cancer

EYES

Test visual acuity in each eye.	Diminished acuity
Assess visual fields, if indicated.	Hemianopsia, quadrantic defects

Inspect the

• Position and alignment of eyes	Exophthalmos, strabismus
• Eyebrows	Seborrheic dermatitis
• Eyelids	Sty, chalazion, ectropion, ptosis, xanthelasma
• Lacrimal apparatus	Swollen lacrimal sac
• Conjunctiva and sclera	Red eye, jaundice
• Cornea, iris, and lens	Corneal opacity, cataract

Examine pupils for

• Size, shape, and equality	Miosis, mydriasis, anisocoria

—*Examination Techniques*—	—*Possible Findings*—
• Reactions to light, and, if these are abnormal—	Absent in 3rd nerve paralysis
• The near reaction	Useful in tonic pupils, Argyll Robertson pupils

Assess the extraocular muscles by observing

• The corneal reflections from a midline light	Muscular imbalance
• The six cardinal fields of gaze	Paralytic or nonparalytic strabismus, nystagmus

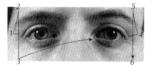

• Convergence	Poor in hyperthyroidism

Inspect the fundi with an ophthalmoscope, including the

• Red reflex	Cataracts, artificial eye
• Optic disc	Papilledema, glaucomatous cupping, optic atrophy

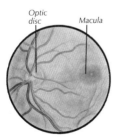

Optic disc   Macula

—Examination Techniques—	—Possible Findings—
• Arteries, veins, and A–V crossings	Hypertensive changes
• Adjacent retina. *Note* any lesions.	Hemorrhages, exudates, cotton-wool patches, microaneurysms, pigmentation
• Macular area	Macular degeneration

——— *The Ears* ———

Examine, on each side,

THE AURICLE

Inspect it.	Keloid, sebaceous cyst

If you suspect otitis,

• **Move the auricle** up and down, and press on the tragus.	Causes pain in otitis externa
• **Press** firmly behind the ear.	May be tender in otitis media and mastoiditis

THE EAR CANAL AND EARDRUM

Pull the auricle up, back, and slightly out.

Inspect, through an otoscope speculum,

• The canal	Cerumen, otitis externa
• The eardrum, as illustrated on the next page	Acute otitis media, serous otitis media, tympanosclerosis, perforations

—Examination Techniques—   *—Possible Findings—*

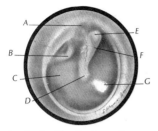

A = Pars flaccida   B = Incus   C = pars
tensa   D = Umbo   E = Short process of
malleus   F = Handle of malleus   G
= Cone of light

(After Hawke M, Keene M, Alberti PW: Clinical Otoscopy: A Text and Colour Atlas. Edinburgh, Churchill Livingstone, 1984)

HEARING

Assess auditory acuity to the whispered or spoken voice.

If hearing is diminished, use a 512-Hz tuning fork to

- **Test** lateralization (**Weber test**)

- **Compare** air and bone conduction (**Rinne test**)

These tests help to distinguish between sensorineural and conduction hearing loss.

——— Nose and Sinuses ———

Inspect the external nose.

Inspect, with a nasal speculum, the

- Nasal mucosa that covers the septum and turbinates, noting its color and any swelling

Swollen and red in viral rhinitis, swollen and pale in allergic rhinitis

—Examination Techniques—	*—Possible Findings—*
• Nasal septum for position and integrity	Deviation, perforation
Palpate the sinuses for tenderness:	Tender in acute sinusitis
• Frontal	
• Maxillary	

————— *Mouth and Pharynx* —————

Inspect the

• Lips	Cyanosis, pallor, cheilosis
• Buccal mucosa	Canker sores
• Gums	Gingivitis, periodontal disease
• Teeth	Dental caries, tooth loss
• Roof of the mouth	Torus palatinus
• Tongue, including	
Papillae	Glossitis
Symmetry	12th cranial nerve paralysis
Any lesions	Cancer of tongue
• Pharynx, including	
Color or any exudate	Pharyngitis
Symmetry of the soft palate as patient says "ah"	10th cranial nerve paralysis

—Examination Techniques—   *—Possible Findings—*

—————— *Neck* ——————————————

Inspect the neck.   Scars, masses, torticollis

Palpate the lymph nodes.   Cervical lymphadenopathy

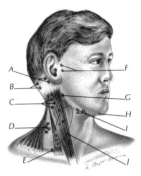

A = Posterior auricular   B = Occipital   C = Superficial cervical   D = Posterior cervical   E = Supraclavicular   F = Preauricular   G = Tonsillar   H = Submental   I = Submaxillary   J = Deep cervical chain

Inspect and **palpate** the   Deviated trachea
position of the trachea.

Inspect the thyroid gland.   Goiter, nodules

• At rest

• As patient swallows water

From behind patient, **pal-**   Goiter, nodules, tenderness
pate the thyroid gland, in-   of thyroiditis
cluding the isthmus and
the lateral lobes, as illustrated on the next page.

—Examination Techniques—   *—Possible Findings—*

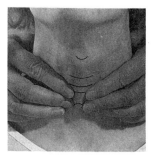

FEELING THE ISTHMUS

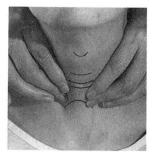

FEELING THE LATERAL LOBES

- At rest

- As patient swallows water

The initial survey of respiration may be done while examining the front of the neck. The musculoskeletal examination of the neck and the upper back and a check for costovertebral angle tenderness may be done after feeling the thyroid gland from behind. The musculoskeletal examination of the upper extremities may be done next or deferred until later.

—Examination Techniques—   *—Possible Findings—*

SPECIAL MANEUVERS

℥   *EVERSION OF THE UPPER EYELID.* The patient should relax and look down.

Grasp eyelashes of upper lid and pull them gently down and forward.

Place an applicator stick or the edge of a tongue blade horizontally on upper lid at least 1 cm above lid margin, and push it down on eyelid, thus everting lid.

Hold lashes of upper lid against eyebrow while you inspect the palpebral conjunctiva.

When finished, pull eyelashes gently forward, and ask patient to look up.

♀/♂ *TRANSILLUMINATION OF THE FRONTAL AND MAXILLARY SINUSES.* In a fully darkened room, shine a bright narrow light

• Upward under each brow. Shield light with your hand and observe forehead.

• Downward from just below the inner aspect of

Eversion of lid reveals foreign bodies and lesions of the palpebral conjunctiva of upper lid.

A local red glow in the forehead or in the roof of the mouth suggests that the frontal or maxillary sinus, respectively, is air-filled. Absence of a glow suggests a thickened mucosa or secretions.

—*Examination Techniques*—	—*Possible Findings*—

each eye. Patient's head should be tilted back, with mouth open. Observe roof of mouth.

─────── *The Thorax and Lungs* ───────

₽ SURVEY

Inspect the thorax and its respiratory movements. *Note*

• Rate, rhythm, depth, and effort of breathing	Tachypnea, hyperpnea, Cheyne-Stokes breathing
• Any retractions of the supraclavicular areas or contractions of the sternomastoid or other muscles on inspiration	Inspiratory muscle contractions indicate impaired lung function.
Observe shape of patient's chest.	Normal or barrel chest
Listen to patient's breathing for	Increased white noise and wheezes in chronic bronchitis and asthma
• Increased white noise	
• Wheezes	

THE POSTERIOR CHEST

Inspect the chest for

• Deformities or asymmetry	Kyphoscoliosis
• Abnormal inspiratory retractions of the interspaces	Retractions in airway obstruction

—Examination Techniques—	*—Possible Findings—*
• Impairment or unilateral lag in respiratory movements	Disease of the underlying lung or pleura

Palpate the chest for

• Tender areas	Fractured ribs
• Assessment of visible abnormalities	Masses, sinus tracts
• Respiratory expansion	Impairment, one or both sides
• Tactile fremitus	Local or generalized decrease or increase

Percuss the chest in the areas illustrated, comparing one side with the other at each level.	Dullness occurs when fluid or solid tissue replaces normally air-filled lung. Hyperresonance often accompanies emphysema or pneumothorax.

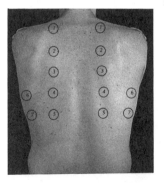

Identify level of diaphragmatic dullness on each side and *estimate* diaphragmatic excursion.	Pleural effusion or a paralyzed diaphragm raises level of dullness.

| *—Examination Techniques—* | *—Possible Findings—* |

Listen to chest with stethoscope in areas shown above, again comparing sides.

- **Evaluate** the breath sounds.

  Vesicular, bronchovesicular, or bronchial breath sounds

- **Note** any adventitious (added) sounds.

  Crackles (fine and coarse) and continuous sounds (wheezes and rhonchi)

Observe their qualities, place in the respiratory cycle, and location on the chest wall. Do they clear with deep breathing or coughing?

Assess transmitted voice sounds if you have heard bronchial breath sounds in abnormal places. Ask patient to

- Say "99" and "ee"

  Bronchophony, egophony, and whispered pectoriloquy

- Whisper "99" or "1, 2, 3"

Inspection of the breasts, examination of the axillae, and palpation of the epitrochlear nodes may be done next while the patient is still sitting. Palpation of a woman's breasts is done after she lies down.

—Examination Techniques—   *—Possible Findings—*

o— THE ANTERIOR CHEST

Inspect the chest for

- Deformities or asymmetry   Pectus excavatum

- Intercostal retractions   From obstructed airways

- Impaired or lagging re-   From disease of the under-
  spiratory movements   lying lung or pleura

Palpate the chest for

- Tender areas   Tender pectoral muscles or
                                 costal cartilages

- Assessment of visible abnormalities

- Respiratory expansion

- Tactile fremitus

Percuss the chest in the   Normal cardiac dullness
areas illustrated.   may disappear in emphy-
                                 sema.

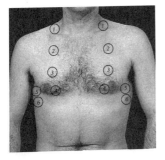

Identify upper border of   May be displaced down-
liver dullness in midclavic-   ward in emphysema
ular line.

—Examination Techniques—   *—Possible Findings—*

Listen to chest with stethoscope. **Note**

- Breath sounds

- Adventitious sounds

- If indicated, transmitted voice sounds

SPECIAL MANEUVERS

⌐ *ASSESSMENT OF PULMONARY FUNCTION*

If appropriate, *walk with patient* down the hall or up a flight of stairs. Observe rate, effort, and sound of breathing, and inquire about symptoms.

⌐ Measure *forced expiratory time.* Ask patient to take a deep breath in and then breathe out as quickly and completely as possible, with mouth open. Listen over trachea with stethoscope and time audible expiration. It should last less than 5 sec. Try to get three consistent readings, allowing rests as necessary.

If the patient understands and cooperates well, a forced expiratory time of > 6 sec strongly suggests obstructive pulmonary disease.

⌐ *IDENTIFICATION OF A FRACTURED RIB.* With one hand on patient's ster-

An increase in local rib pain, distant from your hands, suggests rib fracture

—*Examination Techniques*—   —*Possible Findings*—

num and the other on the thoracic spine, squeeze patient's chest. Does this anteroposterior compression cause pain? If so, where?

rather than just soft-tissue injury.

——— *The Breasts and Axillae* ———

FEMALE BREASTS

Inspect the breasts for

- Size and symmetry

Development, asymmetry

- Contour

Flattening, dimpling

- Appearance of the skin

Edema (peau d'orange)

Inspect the nipples.

- Compare their size and shape.

Inversion, retraction, deviation

- Note any rashes, ulcerations, or discharge.

Paget's disease of the nipple, galactorrhea

Continue your inspection as patient

- Raises both arms above her head

Dimpling and abnormalities of contour

- Presses her hands against her hips

∘— **Palpate** the breasts for

- Consistency

Physiologic nodularity

- Tenderness

Infection, premenstrual tenderness

—*Examination Techniques*—	—*Possible Findings*—
• Nodules. If present, *note* their	Cyst, fibroadenoma, cancer
Location	
Size	
Shape	
Consistency	
Delimitation	
Tenderness	
Mobility	
Palpate each nipple.	Thickening in cancer
Compress each nipple and areola for discharge.	Galactorrhea or discharge from local breast disease

♀/♂—MALE BREASTS

Inspect the nipple and areola.	Gynecomastia, cancer
Palpate the areola and adjacent area.	Gynecomastia, cancer

♀ AXILLAE

Inspect for rashes, infection, and pigmentation.	Hidradenitis suppurativa, acanthosis nigricans
Palpate the central axillary nodes.	Lymphadenopathy

If indicated, **palpate** the other axillary nodes:

• Pectoral group

—Examination Techniques—   *—Possible Findings—*

- Lateral group

- Subscapular group

——————— *The Cardiovascular System* ———————

ᖶ *THE ARTERIAL PULSE*

RADIAL PULSE

Palpate the radial pulse.
Note

- Heart rate   Tachycardia, bradycardia

- Rhythm. If this is irregu-   Premature contractions,
  lar, listen to the heart.   atrial fibrillation

CAROTID ARTERY PULSE

Palpate the carotid artery
pulse. *Note*

- Amplitude   Increased, decreased

- Any variations in ampli-   Pulsus alternans
  tude

- Contour   Rapid upstroke and fall in
                                     aortic regurgitation

- Any thrills. If one is pres-   Aortic stenosis, partial ca-
  ent, listen with a stetho-   rotid obstruction
  scope for a bruit.

BLOOD PRESSURE

Estimate systolic blood   Without this step, an aus-
pressure by palpation and   cultatory gap may be
add 30 mm Hg. Use this   missed.
sum as the target for fur-
ther cuff inflations.

—Examination Techniques—	—Possible Findings—

Measure blood pressure with a sphygmomanometer.

If indicated, check it o—ᕂᕠ.   Orthostatic (postural) hypotension

JUGULAR VEINS

Identify the jugular venous pulsations and their highest point in the neck. Adjust height of bed as necessary.

Measure jugular venous pressure—the vertical distance between this highest point and the sternal angle, normally less than 3 cm to 4 cm.

Elevated venous pressure in right-sided heart failure

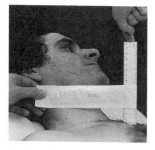

Study the venous pulse waves.   Increased *a* or *v* waves

THE HEART

Inspect and **palpate** the anterior chest for pulsations.

Identify the apical impulse. Turn patient to left as necessary. **Note**

—Examination Techniques—	*—Possible Findings—*
• Location of impulse	Displaced to left in pregnancy; increased diameter, amplitude, and duration in left ventricular enlargement
• Diameter	
• Amplitude	
• Duration	

Feel for an S_3 or S_4.

Feel for a right ventricular impulse in left parasternal and epigastric areas.	Signs of right ventricular enlargement
Palpate left and right second interspaces close to sternum. **Note** any thrills in these areas.	Pulsations of great vessels; accentuated S_2; thrills of aortic or pulmonic stenosis

Listen to heart with stethoscope. Use its diaphragm in all areas illustrated and its bell at the apex and the lower left sternal border.

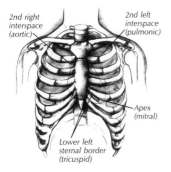

2nd right interspace (aortic)

2nd left interspace (pulmonic)

Apex (mitral)

Lower left sternal border (tricuspid)

Listen at each area

• To S_1

—Examination Techniques—	—Possible Findings—
• To S_2. Is splitting normal in left 2nd and 3rd interspaces?	Physiologic (inspiratory) or pathologic (expiratory) splitting
• For extra sounds in systole	Midsystolic clicks
• For extra sounds in diastole	S_3, S_4
• For systolic murmurs	Midsystolic, pansystolic, late systolic murmurs
• For diastolic murmurs	Early, mid-, or late diastolic murmurs
Identify, if murmurs are present, their	
• Place in cardiac cycle	
• Shape	Plateau, crescendo, decrescendo
• Location of maximal intensity	
• Radiation	
• Intensity on a 6-point scale	
• Pitch	High, medium, low
• Quality	Blowing, harsh, musical, rumbling
❧ **Listen** at the apex with patient turned toward left side.	Left-sided S_3, S_4, and murmur of mitral stenosis

—Examination Techniques—   *—Possible Findings—*

♪ **Listen** down left sternal border to the apex as patient sits, leaning forward, with breath held in exhalation.

Murmur of aortic regurgitation

SPECIAL MANEUVER

↶ *PULSUS ALTERNANS.* Feel pulse for alternation in amplitude. Lower pressure of the blood pressure cuff slowly to systolic level while you listen with a stethoscope over the brachial artery.

Alternating amplitude of pulse or sudden doubling of Korotkoff sounds indicates a pulsus alternans— a sign of left ventricular failure.

↶ *PARADOXICAL PULSE.* Lower pressure of blood pressure cuff slowly toward and past systolic pressure and listen for an absence of sounds during inspiration. Note pressures at which Korotkoff sounds are first heard and at which the sounds persist through the respiratory cycle. These levels are normally not more than 3–4 mm Hg apart.

A difference greater than 10 mm Hg signifies a paradoxical pulse. Consider obstructive lung disease, pericardial tamponade, or constrictive pericarditis.

THE ABDOMINO-JUGULAR TEST. Place bladder of blood pressure cuff on patient's abdomen and inflate bladder with six full squeezes of the bulb. With palm and fingers of one hand, compress pa-

A rise in JVP followed by an abrupt fall of at least 4 cm at time of release suggests heart failure, most often left-sided but at times right-sided.

—Examination Techniques—   *—Possible Findings—*

tient's abdomen through
this bladder for 10 sec at a
pressure level of about 20
mm Hg. Patient should
breathe easily. Note any
change in jugular venous
pressure (JVP). A transient
rise or no rise is normal.

↘/↑ *SQUATTING AND
STANDING.* In suspected
mitral valve prolapse, listen
for the click and murmur in
both positions.

Squatting delays the click
and murmur. Standing re-
verses the changes.

Try to distinguish *aortic stenosis (AS)* from *hypertrophic
cardiomyopathy (HC)* by lis-
tening to the murmur in
both positions.

Squatting increases mur-
mur of AS and decreases
murmur of HC. Standing
reverses the changes.

———— *The Abdomen* ————

○— **Inspect** the abdomen,
including

- Skin

Scars, striae, veins

- Umbilicus

Hernia, inflammation

- Contours for shape, symmetry, enlarged organs or
  masses

Bulging flanks, suprapubic
bulge, large liver or spleen,
tumors

- Any peristaltic waves

GI obstruction

- Any pulsations

Increased in aortic aneu-
rysm

Auscultate the abdomen,
as clinically indicated, for

—Examination Techniques—	*—Possible Findings—*
• Bowel sounds	Increased or decreased motility
• Bruits	Bruit of renal artery stenosis

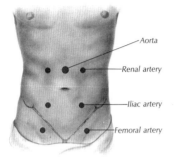

Aorta

Renal artery

Iliac artery

Femoral artery

| • Friction rubs | Liver tumor, splenic infarct |

Percuss the abdomen for

| • Proportions and patterns of tympany and dullness | Ascites, GI obstruction |
| • Span of liver dullness | Hepatomegaly |

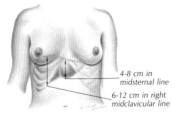

4-8 cm in midsternal line

6-12 cm in right midclavicular line

| • Splenic dullness | Splenomegaly |

—*Examination Techniques*—   —*Possible Findings*—

Palpate all quadrants of
the abdomen

- Lightly for guarding and   Peritoneal inflammation
  tenderness

- Deeply for masses or ten-   Tumors, a distended viscus
  derness

Try, as the patient breathes
in, to **feel** the

- Liver   Hepatomegaly, tender liver
                                    of hepatitis or congestive
                                    heart failure

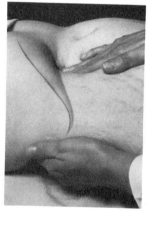

If you cannot feel the
liver with the hand posi-
tions shown, try the
"hooking technique":
hook the fingers of both
hands below the right
costal margin.

—Examination Techniques—   *—Possible Findings—*

• Spleen   Splenomegaly

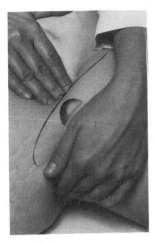

• Kidneys   Enlargement from cysts,
                                      cancer, hydronephrosis;
                                      tenderness from pyelone-
                                      phritis

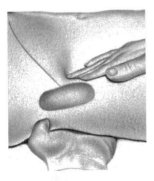

As the patient lies quietly,
palpate the

—Examination Techniques—   *—Possible Findings—*

Abdominal aorta   Aortic aneurysm

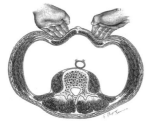 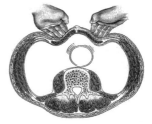

Check for costoverte-
bral angle tenderness.

Tender in kidney infection

SPECIAL MANEUVERS

o— *REBOUND TENDER-
NESS.* Press slowly on a
tender area, then quickly
withdraw your hand.
Greater pain with with-
drawal is rebound tender-
ness.

Rebound tenderness sug-
gests peritoneal inflammation.

o— *SHIFTING DULLNESS
IN ASCITES.* By percus-
sion, map areas of tympany
and dullness with patient
supine and lying on side.

Ascitic fluid usually shifts
to dependent side.

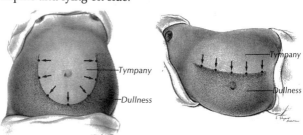

—Examination Techniques—   *—Possible Findings—*

∘— *FLUID WAVE IN ASCITES.* Ask patient or an assistant to press edges of both hands into midline of abdomen. Tap one side, and feel for a wave transmitted to the other side.

A palpable wave suggests but does not prove ascites.

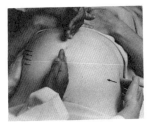

∘— *BALLOTTEMENT.* To find an organ or mass in an ascitic abdomen, try to ballotte it. Place your stiffened and straightened fingers on the abdomen, briefly jab them toward the structure, and try to touch its surface.

Your hand, quickly displacing the fluid, stops abruptly as it touches the solid surface.

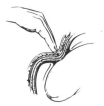

∘— *ASSESSING POSSIBLE APPENDICITIS,* the basic approach:

In classic appendicitis:

"Where did the pain begin?"

Near the umbilicus

—Examination Techniques—	*—Possible Findings—*
"Where is it now?"	Right lower quadrant
Ask patient to cough. Where does it hurt?	Right lower quadrant
Search for local tenderness.	RLQ tenderness
Feel for muscular rigidity.	RLQ rigidity
Perform a rectal exam and, in women, a pelvic exam also.	Possibly local tenderness
○— *MURPHY'S SIGN FOR ACUTE CHOLECYS-TITIS.* Hook your thumb under right costal margin at edge of rectus muscle, and ask patient to take a deep breath.	Sharp tenderness and a sudden stop in inspiratory effort constitutes a positive test.

——— *Male Genitalia* ———

This examination is usually deferred until the patient is standing.

THE PENIS

Inspect the

• Development of the penis and the skin and hair at its base	Sexual maturation, lice
• Prepuce	Phimosis
• Glans	Balanitis, chancre, herpes, warts, cancer

—*Examination Techniques*—	—*Possible Findings*—
• Urethral meatus	Hypospadias, discharge of urethritis

Palpate

• Any visible lesions (with gloves)	Chancre, cancer
• The shaft	Urethral stricture or cancer

THE SCROTUM AND ITS CONTENTS

Inspect

• Contours of scrotum	Hernia, hydrocele, cryptor-chidism
• Skin of scrotum	Rashes

Palpate each

• Testis, noting any	
Lumps	Cancer
Tenderness	Orchitis, torsion
• Epididymis	Epididymitis, cyst
• Spermatic cord and adjacent areas	Varicocele

HERNIAS

Inspect inguinal and femoral areas as patient strains down.	Inguinal and femoral hernias
Palpate external inguinal ring through scrotal skin, and ask patient to strain down.	Indirect and direct inguinal hernias

—Examination Techniques—　　　*—Possible Findings—*

SPECIAL MANEUVER

TRANSILLUMINATION OF A SCROTAL MASS

Darken room, and shine beam of a good flashlight from behind scrotum through mass. Note whether mass lights up with a red glow.

Fluid-filled masses such as cysts light up; those containing blood or solid tissue do not.

--- *Anus, Rectum, and Prostate—Male* ---

Inspect the

- Sacrococcygeal area

  Pilonidal cyst or sinus

- Perianal area

  Hemorrhoids, warts, herpes, chancre, cancer

Palpate the anal canal and rectum with a lubricated and gloved finger. Feel the

- Walls of the rectum

  Cancer of the rectum, polyps

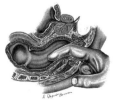

- Prostate gland, as shown on the next page

  Benign hyperplasia, cancer, acute prostatitis

—Examination Techniques—   *—Possible Findings—*

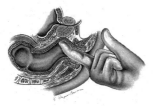

Try to feel above the prostate for irregularities or tenderness, if indicated.

Rectal shelf of peritoneal metastases; tenderness of inflammation

Female Genitalia, Anus, and Rectum

EXTERNAL GENITALIA

o— **Observe** pubic hair to assess sexual maturity.

Normal or delayed puberty

ᴧᴧ **Inspect** the

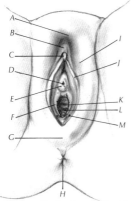

A = Mons pubis   B = Prepuce   C = Clitoris
D = Urethral orifice   E = Opening of Skene's
gland   F = Vestibule   G = Perineum   H
= Anus   I = Labium majus   J = Labium
minus   K = Hymen   L = Vagina   M
= Opening of Bartholin's gland

—*Examination Techniques*—	—*Possible Findings*—
• Labia	Inflammation
• Clitoris	Enlarged in masculinization
• Urethral orifice	Urethral caruncle
• Introitus	Imperforate hymen
Palpate for enlargement or tenderness of Bartholin's glands.	Bartholin's gland infection
Milk the urethra for discharge, if indicated.	Discharge of urethritis

INTERNAL EXAMINATION

Locate the cervix with a gloved and water-lubricated index finger.

Assess support of vaginal outlet by asking patient to strain down.

Cystocele, cystourethrocele, rectocele

Insert a water-lubricated speculum of suitable size, starting with blades held obliquely.

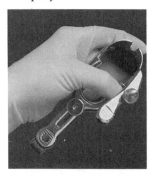

—*Examination Techniques*—	—*Possible Findings*—

Rotate speculum, open blades, and inspect cervix.

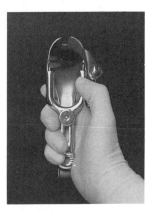

Observe

- Position — Faces forward if uterus is retroverted

- Color — Purplish in pregnancy

- Epithelial surface — Squamous and columnar epithelium

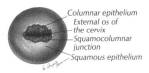

Columnar epithelium
External os of the cervix
Squamocolumnar junction
Squamous epithelium

- Any discharge or bleeding — Mucopurulent cervicitis

- Any ulcers, nodules, or masses — Herpes, polyp, cancer

—*Examination Techniques*—	—*Possible Findings*—
Obtain specimens for cytology (Pap smears) with	Early cancer before it is clinically evident
• An endocervical swab or special brush	
• A spatula to scrape the ectocervix	
Inspect the vaginal mucosa as you withdraw the speculum.	
Palpate, by means of a bimanual examination,	
• The uterus	Pregnancy, myomas
• Right and left adnexa	Ovarian masses, salpingitis, tubal pregnancy
Assess strength of pelvic muscles. With your vaginal fingers clear of the cervix, ask patient to tighten her muscles around your fingers as hard and long as she can.	A firm squeeze that compresses your fingers, moves them up and inward, and lasts more than 3 seconds is full strength.
Perform a rectovaginal examination.	Retroverted uterus

ANUS AND RECTUM

Inspect and **palpate** the anus. Palpate the rectum.	Hemorrhoids, rectal cancer; normal uterine cervix or tampon (felt through rectal wall)

—*Examination Techniques*—   —*Possible Findings*—

—————— *The Peripheral Vascular System* ——————

> Inspection of the limbs may also include findings relevant to the musculoskeletal and nervous systems.

ARMS

Inspect for

• Size and symmetry, any swelling	Lymphedema, venous obstruction
• Venous pattern	
• Color and texture of skin and nails	Raynaud's disease

Palpate the pulses: Lost in thromboangiitis obliterans or acute arterial occlusion

• Radial

• Brachial

Feel for the epitrochlear   Lymphadenopathy
nodes.

LEGS

Inspect for

• Size and symmetry, any swelling	Venous insufficiency, lymphedema
• Venous pattern	Varicose veins

—*Examination Techniques*—	—*Possible Findings*—
• Color and texture of skin	Pallor, rubor, cyanosis
• Hair distribution	Loss in arterial insufficiency
Check for pitting edema.	Peripheral or systemic causes of edema
Palpate the pulses:	Loss of pulses in acute arterial occlusion and arteriosclerosis obliterans
• Femoral	
• Popliteal	
• Dorsalis pedis	
• Posterior tibial	
Palpate the inguinal lymph nodes:	Lymphadenopathy

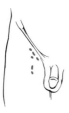

• Horizontal group	
• Vertical group	
Ask patient to stand, and reinspect the venous pattern.	Varicose veins

—Examination Techniques—   *—Possible Findings—*

SPECIAL MANEUVERS

℉ THE MANUAL COM-
PRESSION TEST FOR
COMPETENCY OF
VENOUS VALVES IN
VARICOSE VEINS. Place
one hand on the dilated
vein. At a point at least 20
cm above, compress the
vein firmly with your other
hand. Feel for an impulse
in your lower hand.

An impulse indicates in-
competence of venous
valve(s) between your two
hands.

℉ EVALUATING
ARTERIAL SUPPLY TO
HAND

Feel ulnar pulse, if possible.

Perform an **Allen test.** Ask
patient to make a tight fist,
palm up. Occlude both ra-
dial and ulnar arteries with
your thumbs. Ask patient
to open hand into a re-
laxed, slightly flexed position. Release your pressure
over one artery. Palm
should flush within about 3
to 5 seconds. Repeat, re-
leasing other artery.

Persisting pallor of palm
indicates occlusion of the
released artery or its distal
branches.

o—/℉POSTURAL COLOR
CHANGES OF CHRONIC
ARTERIAL INSUFFI-
CIENCY. Raise both legs to
about 60° for about a min-
ute. Then ask patient to sit
up with legs dangling
down. Note time required

Marked pallor of feet on
elevation, delayed color return and venous filling,
and rubor of dependent
feet suggest arterial insufficiency.

—Examination Techniques—   *—Possible Findings—*

for (1) return of pinkness,
normally about 10 sec or
less, and (2) filling of veins
on feet and ankles, nor-
mally about 15 sec. Watch
for development of any un-
usual rubor.

The Musculoskeletal System

Screening

Inspect the joints and
surrounding tissues as
you examine the various
parts of the body.

Observe:

- Ease and range of mo-
  tion

- Any signs of inflam-
  mation in or around
  joints

- Condition of sur-
  rounding tissues

- Any musculoskeletal
  deformities, including
  abnormal curvatures
  of the spine

Assess the spine, especially during adoles-
cence.

Asymptomatic scoliosis
often becomes evident
in adolescence.

Outlined below is an examination appropriate to a patient with joint symptoms.

—Examination Techniques—   *—Possible Findings—*

ᖯ HEAD AND NECK

Palpate the temporomandibular joint as patient opens and closes mouth.

Swelling, tenderness, and decreased motion in arthritis

Inspect the neck for deformities.

Torticollis, ankylosing spondylitis

Palpate the cervical spine and muscles from behind patient.

Local tenderness

Test the range of neck motion in

- Flexion

- Extension

- Rotation

- Lateral bending

HANDS AND WRISTS

Ask patient to

- Make a fist with each hand

Consider functional significance of limited motion.

- Straighten fingers

- Flex and extend wrists

- Turn hands (with palms down) laterally and medially (lateral and medial deviation)

Inspect hands and wrists.

Deformities, swelling, muscular atrophy

—Examination Techniques—	*—Possible Findings—*

Palpate

- Distal and proximal interphalangeal joints

Proximal joint swelling in
rheumatoid arthritis; nodules of osteoarthritis

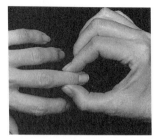

- Metacarpophalangeal
  joints

Swelling in rheumatoid arthritis

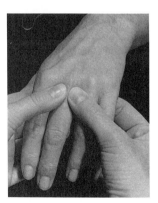

- Wrist joints, as illustrated
  on the next page

Wrist swelling in rheuma-
toid arthritis and in gonococcal infection of the joint
or tendon sheath

—Examination Techniques—   *—Possible Findings—*

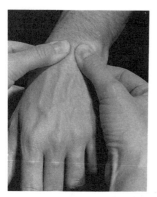

ELBOWS

Ask patient to

- Bend and straighten elbows

- Turn palms up and down (supination and pronation of forearms)

Inspect and **palpate** the elbows, including the

• Olecranon process	Olecranon bursitis
• Grooves overlying the elbow joint	Tenderness in arthritis
• Medial and lateral epicondyles	Tender in epicondylitis
• Extensor surface of the ulna	Rheumatoid nodules

—*Examination Techniques*—   —*Possible Findings*—

SHOULDERS

Ask patient to

- Raise both arms vertically

- Place both hands behind neck with elbows out (abduction and external rotation)

- Place both hands behind small of back (internal rotation)

Consider functional significance to patient when these or other movements are limited.

Inspect shoulders and shoulder girdles from front and back.

Muscular atrophy

Palpate for tenderness, including areas illustrated.

Rotator cuff tendinitis is the most common cause of subacromial tenderness.

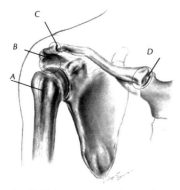

A = *Bicipital groove*   B = *Subacromial area*   C = *Acromioclavicular joint*   D = *Sternoclavicular joint*

—Examination Techniques—   *—Possible Findings—*

⊶ ANKLES AND FEET

Inspect ankles and feet.   Hallux valgus, corns, calluses

Palpate ankle joints.   Tender joint in arthritis; tender ligaments in a sprain

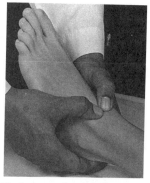

Feel along the Achilles tendons.   Rheumatoid nodules

Squeeze each forefoot, thus compressing the metatarsophalangeal joints; then   Tenderness in arthritis and other conditions

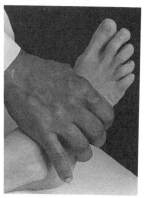

—Examination Techniques—	*—Possible Findings—*

palpate each joint between
your thumb and finger.

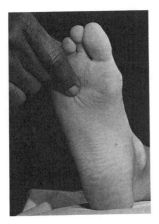

Assess range of motion.	An arthritic joint often hurts when moved in any direction. A sprain hurts chiefly when the injured ligament is stretched.
• Dorsiflex and plantar flex foot at ankle (tibiotalar joint).	

—Examination Techniques—   *—Possible Findings—*

- Stabilize ankle with one
  hand and invert and
  evert heel (subtalar joint).

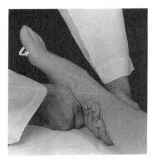

INVERSION

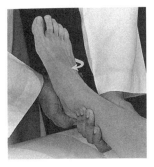

EVERSION

—Examination Techniques—   *—Possible Findings—*

- Stabilize heel and invert and evert forefoot (transverse tarsal joint).

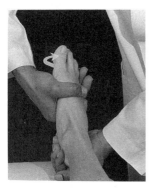

INVERSION

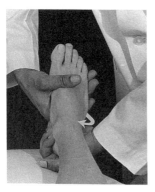

EVERSION

- Flex toes at metatarsophalangeal joints.

—Examination Techniques—   *—Possible Findings—*

KNEES AND HIPS

Inspect and **palpate** each   Bowlegs, knock-knees
knee, including the

- Area of the suprapatellar   Swelling above and beside
  pouch   patella suggests joint fluid.

- Hollow on each side of
  the patella

- Patella   Swelling of prepatellar bur-
                                     sitis

Assess the patellofemoral
compartment.

- Pressing on patella, move
  it against underlying   Pain and crepitus on both
  femur.   maneuvers may occur in
                                 osteoarthritis and chondro-
                                 malacia patellae.

- Push patella distally and
  ask patient to tighten
  knee against table.

With patient's knee flexed   Tenderness of an injured
to 90°, **palpate** the tibio-   prepatellar fat pad or in-
femoral joint.   jured meniscus

Patella
Lateral epicondyle
Patellar tendon
Lateral collateral ligament
Tibia
Tibial tuberosity

—Examination Techniques—	*—Possible Findings—*

Check range of motion, including

- Flexion at hip and knee

Flexion of opposite leg suggests a flexion deformity of that hip.

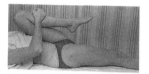

- Rotation at hip, both external (shown below) and internal

Restricted in hip disease

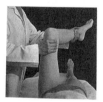

- Abduction at hip

Restricted in hip disease

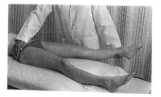

Observe any deformities of knees or feet when patient stands.

Popliteal swelling of a Baker's cyst, flat feet

—*Examination Techniques*—   —*Possible Findings*—

♀ THE SPINE

Inspect spine from side and back, noting any abnormal curvatures. Look for any asymmetries of shoulders, iliac crests, or buttocks.

Kyphosis, scoliosis, lordosis, gibbus, list

Pelvic tilt

Check range of motion in

- Flexion. Watch for normal flattening of lumbar curve.

Persisting lumbar concavity and decreased range of motion due to muscle spasm, disc disease, or ankylosing spondylitis

- Lateral bending

- Extension

- Rotation

Palpate for tenderness of the

Tenderness from disc disease, muscle spasm, compression fracture and other conditions

- Spinous processes

- Paravertebral muscles

SPECIAL MANEUVERS

♀ *PHALEN'S TEST FOR CARPAL TUNNEL SYNDROME.* Hold patient's wrists in acute flexion, or ask patient to press backs of both hands together to form right angles. Either position should be held for 60 seconds.

Numbness or tingling over distribution of median nerve is a positive sign, suggesting carpal tunnel syndrome.

—Examination Techniques—   *—Possible Findings—*

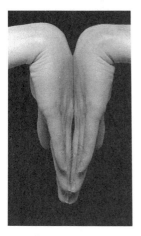

PHALEN'S TEST

⌐
╵   *TINEL'S SIGN FOR
CARPAL TUNNEL SYN-
DROME.* Percuss lightly
over median nerve at wrist.

Tingling or electric sensations in distribution of median nerve is a positive sign.

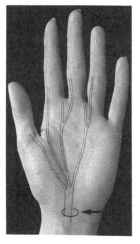

TINEL'S SIGN

—Examination Techniques—   *—Possible Findings—*

○— *THE BULGE SIGN
FOR FLUID IN KNEE
JOINT.* Milk knee upward
to displace any fluid. Then
press behind lateral edge of
patella and watch for re-
turning fluid.

A bulge of returning fluid
indicates fluid within knee
joint. This is a sensitive test
for a small effusion.

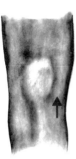

Milk upward

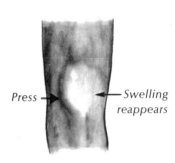

Press →   ← *Swelling
reappears*

○— *BALLOTTEMENT OF
PATELLA FOR FLUID IN
KNEE JOINT.* With one
hand, compress region of
suprapatellar pouch; with
the other, push patella
briskly back against underlying femur.

A palpable click indicates
fluid within knee joint.
This is a good test for a relatively large effusion.

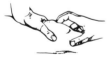

○— *STRAIGHT LEG
RAISING.* Raise patient's
straightened leg until pain
occurs. Then dorsiflex foot.

Sharp pain down back of
leg suggests tension on or
compression of a nerve
root. Dorsiflexion increases
pain.

—Examination Techniques—   *—Possible Findings—*

**○— MEASURING LEG
LENGTH.** Patient's legs
should be aligned symmetrically. With a tape, measure distance from anterior
superior iliac spine to medial malleolus. Tape should
cross knee medially.

Unequal leg length may be
the cause of scoliosis.

**℔/○— MEASURING RANGE
OF MOTION.** To measure
range of motion precisely, a
simple pocket goniometer is
needed. Estimates may be
made visually. Movement
in the elbow at the right is
limited to range indicated
by red lines.

A flexion deformity of 45°
and further flexion to 90°
(45° → 90°).

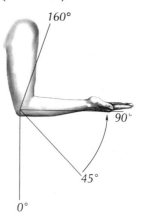

The Nervous System

Screening

CRANIAL NERVES

- N2. Visual acuity, visual fields, ocular
  fundi

—Examination Techniques—   *—Possible Findings—*

- N2, 3. Pupillary reactions

- N3, 4, 6. Extraocular movements

- N5. Corneal reflexes, jaw movements

- N7. Facial movements

- N8. Hearing

- N9, 10. Swallowing, rise of palate, voice

- N12. Appearance of tongue

- N5, 7, 10, 12. Speech

GAIT AND LEGS

- Walk and turn, walk heel-to-toe, walk on toes and on heels.

- Hop in place.

- Do shallow knee bends.

ROMBERG TEST

SHOULDERS, ARMS, AND HANDS

- Pronator drift

- Arm strength with hands overhead

—Examination Techniques—   *—Possible Findings—*

- Winging

- Grip

MOTOR SYSTEM

- Involuntary movements, abnormal positions

- Muscle bulk

- Muscle tone

- Rapid alternating movements in the hands

SENSORY SYSTEM

- Pain sensation in hands and feet

- Vibration sense in hands and feet

- Light touch on arms and legs

- Stereognosis in hands

Outlined below is a more thorough examination of the nervous system.

CRANIAL NERVES

N1 (Olfactory). **Test** sense of smell on each side.   Loss in frontal lobe lesions

—Examination Techniques—   *—Possible Findings—*

N2 (Optic)

Assess visual acuity.   Blindness

Check visual fields.   Hemianopsia

Inspect optic discs.   Papilledema, optic atrophy

N2, 3 (Optic and Oculomo-   Blindness, N3 paralysis,
tor). **Test** pupillary reac-   tonic pupils, Horner's syn-
tions to light. If they are   drome
abnormal, test reactions to
near effort.

N3, 4, and 6 (Oculomotor,   Strabismus from paralysis
Trochlear, and Abducens).   of N3, 4, or 6; nystagmus
Assess extraocular move-
ments.

N5 (Trigeminal)   Motor or sensory loss from
                                     lesions of N5 or its higher
                                     motor pathways

Feel the contractions of
temporal and masseter
muscles.

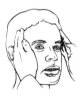

—Examination Techniques—   *—Possible Findings—*

Check corneal reflexes.

Test pain and light touch senses on face.

N7 (Facial). **Ask** patient to raise both eyebrows, frown, close eyes tightly, show teeth, smile, and puff out cheeks.

Weakness in Bell's palsy or from upper motor neuron damage

N8 (Acoustic). **Assess** hearing. If it is decreased—

- **Test** for lateralization (**Weber test**).

- **Compare** air and bone conduction (**Rinne test**).

Sensorineural loss causes lateralization to less affected ear and AC > BC. Conduction loss causes lateralization to more affected ear and BC > AC.

N9 and 10 (Glossopharyngeal and Vagus)

Observe any difficulty in swallowing.

A weakened palate or pharynx impairs swallowing.

Listen to the voice.

Hoarse or nasal voice

Watch soft palate rise with "ah."

Palatal paralysis

Test gag reflex on each side.

Absent reflex

N11 (Spinal Accessory)

—*Examination Techniques*—	—*Possible Findings*—
• Trapezius muscles. **Assess** bulk, involuntary movements, and strength of shoulder shrug.	Atrophy, fasciculations, weakness
• Sternomastoid muscles. **Assess** strength as head turns against your hand.	Weakness

N12 (Hypoglossal).

Listen to patient's articulation.	Dysarthria from damage to N5, 7, 10, or 12
Inspect the resting tongue.	Atrophy, fasciculations
Inspect the protruded tongue.	Deviation to weak side

⌐ NEUROLOGIC SCREENING

Gait and Legs. **Ask** patient to

• Walk away, turn, and come back	Upper or lower motor weakness, cerebellar ataxia, parkinsonism, and loss of position sense may all affect performance.
• Walk heel-to-toe	
• Walk on toes, then on heels	
• Hop in place on each foot	
• Do one-legged shallow knee bends	

(Substitute rising from a chair and climbing on a stool for hops and bends as indicated.)

—*Examination Techniques*—   —*Possible Findings*—

Romberg Test. **Ask** patient to stand with feet together and eyes open, then closed for 20 to 30 seconds. Mild swaying may occur. (Stand close by to prevent falls.)

Loss of balance that appears when eyes are closed is a positive Romberg test, suggesting poor position sense.

Arms, Shoulders, and Hands

Check for a *pronator drift.* Watch as patient holds arms forward, with eyes closed, for 20 to 30 seconds.

Flexion and pronation in hemiplegia

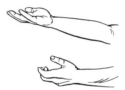

Ask patient to keep arms up, and **tap** them downward. A smooth return to position is normal.

Weakness, incoordination, poor position sense

Test *arm strength* further by asking patient to raise both arms overhead. Try to force them down.

Upper or lower motor neuron weakness

Watch for *winging* as patient lowers both arms slowly forward and down or pushes forward against resistance.

Winging from weakness of the serratus anterior

—Examination Techniques—   *—Possible Findings—*

Test *grip* in each hand.

Weakness from motor deficits or arthritis

THE MOTOR SYSTEM

Involuntary Movements. If movements are present, **observe** their location, quality, rate, rhythm, amplitude, and setting.

Tremors, fasciculations, tics, chorea, athetosis, oral–facial dyskinesias

Muscle Bulk. **Inspect** muscle contours.

Atrophy

🖐/•— *Muscle Tone.* **Assess** resistance to passive stretch of arms and legs.

Spasticity, rigidity, flaccidity

Muscle Strength in major muscle groups:

🖐
- Elbow flexion (C5,6)

- Elbow extension (C6,7,8)

- Wrist extension (C6,7,8, radial nerve)

- Finger abduction (C8, T1, ulnar nerve)

Look for a pattern in any detectable weakness. It may suggest a lower motor lesion affecting a peripheral nerve or nerve root. Weakness of one side of body suggests an upper motor neuron lesion. A polyneuropathy causes symmetrical distal weakness, and a myopathy usually causes proximal weakness. Weakness that worsens with repeated effort and improves with rest suggests myasthenia gravis.

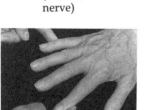

—Examination Techniques—   *—Possible Findings—*

- Thumb opposition (C8, T1, median nerve)

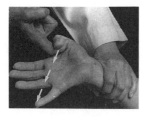

- Trunk

  Flexion, extension, lateral bending

  Thoracic expansion, diaphragmatic excursion

- Hip flexion (L2,3,4)

- Hip abduction (L4,5,S1)

- Hip adduction (L2,3,4)

- Knee extension (L2,3,4)

- Knee flexion (L4,5, S1,2)

- Ankle dorsiflexion (L4,5)

- Ankle plantar flexion (S1)

Scale for Grading Muscle Strength:

0 No muscular contraction detected

1 A barely detectable trace of contraction

2 Active movement with gravity eliminated

3 Active movement against gravity

4 Active movement against gravity and some resistance

5 Active movement against full resistance

 —REFLEXES

- Biceps (C5,6)

Hyperactive deep tendon reflexes, absent abdominal reflexes, and a Babinski response indicate an upper motor neuron lesion. Clonus of the deep tendon reflexes is often associated with hyperactivity.

- Triceps (C6,7)

—Examination Techniques—   *—Possible Findings—*

- Supinator (brachiora-
  dialis) (C5,6)

- Abdominals

  Upper (T8,9,10)

  Lower (T10,11,12)

- Knee (L2,3,4)

- Ankle (S1)

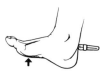

—Examination Techniques—	*—Possible Findings—*

- Plantar (L5, S1), normally flexor

Babinski response

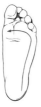
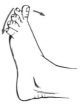

Check for clonus if reflexes are hyperactive

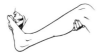

Reinforce absent reflexes by isometric contraction of unrelated muscles.

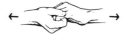

Scale for Grading Reflexes

4+ Hyperactive, often with clonus

3+ Brisker than average, not necessarily abnormal

2+ Average, normal

1+ Diminished, low normal

0 No response

—Examination Techniques—   *—Possible Findings—*

THE SENSORY SYSTEM

Methods of Testing

꿈/o— **Compare** symmetri-   Hemisensory deficits
cal areas on the two sides
of the body.

Also compare distal and   Glove-and-stocking loss of
proximal areas of arms and   peripheral neuropathy
legs for *pain, temperature,*
and touch sensations. Scatter
stimuli to sample most der-
matomes and major pe-
ripheral nerves.

Check fingers and toes dis-   Loss of position and vibra-
tally for *vibration and posi-*   tion senses in posterior col-
tion senses. If responses are   umn disease
abnormal, test more proxi-
mally.

Map out any area of abnormal response.

Except when you are ex-
plaining the tests, patient's
eyes should be closed.

Assess response to the following stimuli:

- *Pain.* Use the sharp end   Analgesia, hypalgesia, hy-
  of a pin or other suitable   peralgesia
  tool. The dull end serves
  as a control.

- *Temperature* (if indicated).   Temperature and pain
  Use test tubes with hot   senses usually correlate
  and ice-cold water (or   with each other.
  other objects of suitable
  temperature).

—*Examination Techniques*—	—*Possible Findings*—

- *Light touch.* Use a fine wisp of cotton.

Anesthesia, hyperesthesia

- *Vibration.* Use a 128-Hz or 256-Hz tuning fork, held on a bony prominence.

Vibration and position senses, both carried in the posterior columns, often correlate with each other.

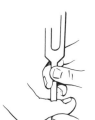

- *Position.* Holding patient's finger or big toe by its sides, move it up or down.

Discriminative Sensations

- *Stereognosis.* **Ask** for identification of a common object placed in patient's hand.

Stereognosis, number identification, and two-point discrimination may be impaired by lesions in the posterior columns or in the sensory cortex.

—Examination Techniques—   *—Possible Findings—*

- *Number identification.*
  Ask for identification of
  a number drawn on pa-
  tient's palm with blunt
  end of a pen.

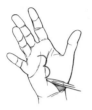

- *Two-point discrimination.*
  Find minimal distance on
  pad of patient's finger at
  which the sides of two
  points can be distin-
  guished from one
  (normally <5 mm).

- *Point localization.* **Touch**
  skin briefly, and **ask** patient to open both eyes
  and identify the place
  touched.

- *Extinction.* Simulta-
  neously **touch** opposite,
  corresponding areas of
  the body, and **ask** patient
  where the touch is felt.

A lesion in the sensory cortex may impair point localization, and stimuli on side
opposite lesion may be ex-
tinguished.

—*Examination Techniques*—   —*Possible Findings*—

SPECIAL MANEUVERS

∘— *MENINGEAL SIGNS.*
With patient supine, flex
head and neck toward
chest. Note resistance or
pain, and watch for flexion
of hips and knees (**Brud-
zinski's sign**).

Meningeal irritation may
cause resistance to and
pain on flexion during both
these maneuvers. A com-
pressed lumbosacral nerve
root also causes pain on
straightening the knee of a
raised leg.

Flex one of patient's legs at
hip and knee, then
straighten knee. Note resistance or pain (**Kernig's
sign**).

ᡂ *ASTERIXIS.* **Ask** the patient to hold both arms forward, with hands cocked
up and fingers spread.
Watch for 1 to 2 minutes.

Sudden brief flexions suggest a metabolic encepha-
lopathy.

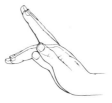

∘— *SPECIAL TESTS FOR
THE STUPOROUS OR
COMATOSE PATIENT*

*Assess response to progres-
sive stimuli:*

• A simple command

• Calling patient's name

• Painful stimuli, such as
  pinching inner, upper
  part of arm or thigh.
  Start gently.

Evidence of motor or sen-
sory loss on one side

—Examination Techniques—   *—Possible Findings—*

Test for flaccid paralysis:

- Hold the forearms vertically and note wrist positions.

  A flaccid hand droops to the horizontal.

- From 12 to 18 inches above bed, drop each arm.

  A flaccid arm drops more rapidly.

- Support both knees in a somewhat flexed position, then extend one knee and let it drop to the bed.

  The flaccid leg drops more rapidly.

- From a similar starting position, release both legs.

  A flaccid leg falls into extension and external rotation.

Check for the oculocephalic reflex (doll's eye movements). Holding upper eyelids open, turn head quickly to each side, then forward in flexion and backward in extension.

In a comatose patient with an intact brainstem, the eyes move in the opposite direction (doll's eye movements).

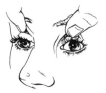 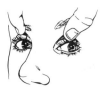

Very deep coma or a lesion in midbrain or pons abolishes this reflex.

3

The Examination of Infants and Children

While most of the techniques used to examine adults are applicable to infants and children, there are methods of examination that are unique during infancy (the first year of life), early childhood (1 through 4 years), and late childhood (5 through 12 years). Those for which there are differences in methodology will be described here, following the outline for each of the sections of Chapter 2, The Physical Examination of an Adult. Where no differences exist, no comment will be made. The physical examination of adolescents (13 through 20 years) is conducted essentially as that of the adult.

Sequence of a Comprehensive Examination

Positions for various parts of the examination during infancy and early childhood need not necessarily follow those recommended for examining adults. Some parts can be conducted on the parent's lap with the baby supine or sitting (or even on your own lap). The supine position on the examining table is essential for examination of the abdomen, hips, genitalia, and rectum, and of the mouth and the ears when the baby is resisting.

—*Examination Techniques*—	—*Possible Findings*—

Infancy and Early Childhood. No special sequence except that oral and ear examination, abduction of the hips, and the rectal examination (if needed) should be saved until last, since these usually cause the baby to cry. Be opportunistic and listen to the heart and lungs and palpate the abdomen when the baby is quiet.

Late Childhood. Use the same order of examination as with adults, except examine the most painful areas last.

——— *Mental and Physical Status* ———

Infancy. Observe the parents' affect in talking about their baby, their manner of holding, moving, and dressing the baby, and their response to situations that may produce discomfort for the baby. Observe a breast or bottle feeding.	Normal parental bonding to the infant. Maladaptive parental nurturing as a cause of malnutrition and "failure to thrive"
Determine attainment of developmental milestones using the Denver Developmental Screening Test before conducting the physical examination.	Normal development *versus* delays in personal-social, fine motor-adaptive, language, and gross motor development

—*Examination Techniques*—	—*Possible Findings*—
Early Childhood. Observe during the interview the degree of sickness or wellness, mood, state of nutrition, speech, cry, facial expression, apparent chronological and emotional age, developmental skills, and parent–child interaction, including the amount of separation tolerance, displays of affection, and response to discipline.	Normal or abnormal level of general health and development. Parents who abuse their children often pay little attention to them; abused children usually demonstrate no anxiety when separated from their parents.
Late Childhood. Determine the child's orientation to time and place, factual knowledge, and language and number skills. Observe motor skills used in writing, tying shoelaces, buttoning, using scissors, and drawing.	Normal or abnormal performance, the latter suggesting intellectual impairment or motor disability

The General Survey

Measurements of vital signs and body size in infants and children often provide the first and only indicators of disease.	Sepsis, chronic renal failure, congenital heart disease, parental deprivation

HEIGHT AND WEIGHT

Growth, reflected in increases in body height and weight within expected limits, is probably the best indicator of health during infancy and childhood. Each child's height and	Growth measures above the 97th or below the 3rd percentile, or if there has been a recent rise or fall from prior levels, require investigation.

—Examination Techniques—   *—Possible Findings—*

weight should be plotted
on standard growth charts
to determine if normal progress is being made. See
standard grids on pp.
117–120.

HEAD CIRCUMFERENCE

Determine the head cir-
cumference at every physical examination during the
first 2 years and at least
biennially thereafter.

Microcephaly, premature
closure of the sutures, hy-
drocephalus, subdural he-
matoma, brain tumor

With the patient supine,
place a cloth, soft plastic, or
disposable paper centimeter
tape over the occipital, pa-
rietal, and frontal promi-
nences of the head.

Individual and/or serial
measurements of the head
circumference are essential
for determination of re-
tarded and overly rapid
growth of the head.

Stretch the tape and note
the reading, being sure that
the greatest circumference
is obtained.

SPECIAL MANEUVER

*FLUSH TECHNIQUE FOR
MEASURING BLOOD
PRESSURE* (In infants and
children <3 years of age).
With the cuff in place,
wrap an elastic bandage
snugly around the elevated
arm, proceeding from
fingers to antecubital space.
Inflate the cuff to a pres-

—*Examination Techniques*—	—*Possible Findings*—
sure above the expected systolic reading.	
Remove the bandage and place the pallid arm at the patient's side. Allow the pressure to fall slowly until the flush of normal color returns to the forearm, hand, and fingers.	When flushing occurs, the sphygmomanometer reading will indicate a blood pressure value somewhere between the systolic and diastolic levels.

THE SKIN

Infancy. Look for

• Pallor	Anoxia, anemia
• Vasomotor changes	Mottled appearance common in prematurity, cretinism, Down's syndrome
• Cyanosis	Acrocyanosis, congenital heart disease
• Melanotic pigmentation	Mongolian spots
• Jaundice	Sepsis, hemolytic disease, biliary obstruction
• Erythema	Miliaria rubra, erythema toxicum, capillary hemangioma, port-wine stain

——— *The Head* ———————

Infancy. Palpate the	Head small with microcephaly, enlarged with hydrocephaly
• Anterior and posterior fontanelles	Fontanelles full and tense with meningitis

—Examination Techniques—	—Possible Findings—
• Sagittal, coronal, and lambdoidal sutures	Closed with microcephaly. Separated with increased intracranial pressure (hydrocephaly, subdural hematoma, and brain tumor).
• Cranial bones	Swelling due to subperiosteal hemorrhage (cephalohematoma) does not cross suture lines; swelling due to bleeding associated with a fracture does.
Early and Late Childhood. Auscultate the skull.	A bruit in a nonanemic child suggests increased intracranial pressure or an intracranial arteriovenous shunt.

SPECIAL MANEUVERS

MACEWEN'S SIGN. Percuss the parietal bone on each side by tapping your index or middle finger directly against its surface.	A "cracked pot" sound is heard prior to closure of the sutures and when increased intracranial pressure causes closed sutures to separate (*e.g.*, in lead encephalopathy and brain tumor).
TRANSILLUMINATION OF THE SKULL. In a completely darkened room, place a standard three-battery flashlight, with a soft rubber collar attached to the lighted end, flush against the skull at various points. Normally, a 2-cm halo of light is present around the circumference	Uniform transillumination of the entire head occurs when the cerebral cortex is partially absent or thinned. Localized bright spots may be seen with subdural effusion and porencephalic cysts.

—Examination Techniques—   *—Possible Findings—*

of the flashlight over the frontoparietal area and a 1-cm halo over the occipital area.

CHVOSTEK'S SIGN. Percuss the top of the cheek just below the zygomatic bone in front of the ear, using the tip of your index or middle finger.

One or two contractions of the facial muscles may occur normally during infancy and early childhood. Repeated contractions occur in tetanus and in tetany due to hypocalcemia and hyperventilation.

———— *The Eyes* ————

Infancy. Test for vision by shining a bright light into the eye or moving an object quickly toward it.

Blinking of the eyes and extension of the head will occur if the baby can see.

Early Childhood. Test for vision in children under 4 years of age by giving the child a set of small toys (*e.g.,* a cube, a marble, a coin). Hold an identical set where the child can see it, at a distance of 10 feet. Pick up each item and ask the child to point to or pick up the matching toy from the child's set.

Failure to match provides only an indication of impaired vision, not the degree of impairment.

SPECIAL MANEUVERS

EXAMINATION OF AN INFANT'S EYES. Hold the baby upright, grasping the

The eyes look in the direction you are turning. When the rotation stops, the eyes

—Examination Techniques—

—Possible Findings—

axillae with your hands and fixing the head with your thumbs. Extend your arms and rotate yourself with the baby slowly in one direction. The baby's eyes will open, providing a clear view of the scleras, irises, and extraocular movements.

look in the opposite direction.

COVER–UNCOVER TEST FOR STRABISMUS. Attract the child's attention to a light held at your midforehead. Place your other hand on top of the child's head and your thumb in front of one eye while observing the other for movement. Remove your thumb and observe both eyes for movement. Repeat the test, covering and uncovering the other eye with your thumb.

If either or both eyes move, a strabismus is present. The eye movements with monocular right esotropia are illustrated below.

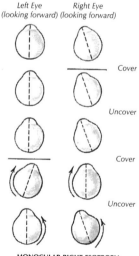

Left Eye
(looking forward)

Right Eye
(looking forward)

Cover

Uncover

Cover

Uncover

MONOCULAR RIGHT ESOTROPIA

—Examination Techniques—   *—Possible Findings—*

———— *The Ears* ————————————

THE AURICLE

Infancy. Note whether the upper portion of the newborn's auricle joins the scalp below a line drawn across the inner canthus and outer canthus of the eye.

Auricles that join the scalp below this line suggest the presence of renal agenesis.

THE EAR CANAL AND EARDRUM

Infancy. Visualize the eardrum with your otoscope by pulling the pinna downward.

The light reflex on the tympanic membrane is diffuse and does not become cone-shaped until several months after birth.

HEARING

Infancy. Make a loud, sharp noise near the infant's ear and watch for blinking of the eyes (**acoustic blink reflex**).

Absence may indicate decreased hearing.

SPECIAL MANEUVER

PNEUMATIC OTOSCOPY. Place the speculum of a pneumatic otoscope far enough into the external ear canal to provide a relatively tight air seal. Introduce or remove air from the canal by applying positive and negative pressures with a rubber squeeze bulb attached to the otoscope, as illustrated on the next page.

When air is introduced the tympanic membrane moves inward, and when air is removed the membrane moves outward. This movement is absent in serous otitis media, and diminished in some cases of acute otitis media.

—Examination Techniques—   *—Possible Findings—*

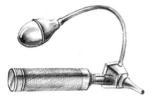

————— *The Nose, Mouth, Pharynx, and Neck* —————

NOSE

Infancy. Test the patency of the nasal passages by occluding each nostril alternately while holding the infant's mouth closed.

The baby will be unable to breathe when choanal atresia is present.

MOUTH

Early and Late Childhood. Ask the child to bite down as hard as possible. Part the lips and observe the alignment of the maxilla and mandible.

Normally, the upper teeth slightly override the lower teeth. Overbite and underbite can be detected this way.

NECK

Infancy. Inspect and palpate the newborn's neck for skin tags, fistulas, masses, cysts, muscle spasm, and crepitus.

Thyroglossal duct fistula or cyst, branchial cleft fistula or cyst, and sternomastoid muscle injury and fractured clavicle from birth trauma

————— *The Thorax and Lungs* —————

Infancy

- Note the breathing pattern.

Alternating rapid (30 to 40/min) and slow (5 to 10/

—*Examination Techniques*—	—*Possible Findings*—
	min) respirations are considered normal ("periodic") breathing. Apnea (>20 sec) with cardiopulmonary or CNS disease or with high risk for Sudden Infant Death Syndrome (SIDS)
• Note head movement with breathing.	Extension of head on inspiration with severe respiratory disease
• Auscultate the chest with the bell or small diaphragm, listening for breath sounds.	Rarely absent, even with atelectasis, effusion, empyema, or pneumothorax. Inspiratory wheeze with narrowing of upper airway, expiratory wheeze with narrowing of lower airway. Fine crackles normally heard at the end of deep inspiration

———— *The Breasts and Axillae* ————

BREASTS

Infancy. Look for enlargement of the newborn's breasts with white discharge from nipples (witch's milk).	Normal maternal estrogenic effect lasting several days
Late Childhood. Look for asymmetry of breast size in females.	Usual during preadolescence

AXILLAE

Early and Late Childhood. Look for freckles.	Often present with neurofibromatosis

—Examination Techniques—   *—Possible Findings—*

The Cardiovascular System

THE ARTERIAL PULSE

Palpate the femoral pulses.

Diminution (as compared to radial pulse) or absence with coarctation of the aorta

BLOOD PRESSURE

See section above under The General Survey for measurement with the flush method and section in Chapter 4 (pp. 149–150) on blood pressure for normal and abnormal levels in children.

THE HEART

Look and palpate for the apical pulse.

At 4th interspace until age 7 years, at 5th interspace thereafter. To left of mid-clavicular line until 4 years, at MCL between 4 and 6 years, and to right of MCL after age 7 years.

The Abdomen

Infancy. Inspect the newborn's umbilical cord.

There should be two thick-walled arteries and one thin-walled vein. A single umbilical artery suggests the presence of a variety of congenital anomalies.

SPECIAL MANEUVERS

EXAMINATION FOR PY-LORIC STENOSIS. Place

With pyloric stenosis, peristaltic waves are seen going

—*Examination Techniques*—

—*Possible Findings*—

the unclothed infant supine and stand at the foot of the examining table. Direct a bright light at table height across the abdomen from the infant's right side. Feed the baby a bottle of sugar water and observe the abdomen closely. After vomiting occurs, palpate deeply in the right upper quadrant with the baby supine and then prone, using your extended middle finger.

across the upper abdomen from left to right with increasing amplitude and frequency until the infant vomits with projectile force. The olive-size hypertrophied pyloric muscle will be felt.

SCRATCH TEST TO DETERMINE LIVER SIZE. Place the diaphragm of your stethoscope just above the right costal margin at the midclavicular line. With your fingernail, lightly scratch the skin of the abdomen along the midclavicular line, moving from below the umbilicus towards the costal margin. Listen for the sound of the scratching.

When the fingernail reaches the liver's lower edge, the sound of scratching will first be heard as it is transmitted through the liver.

——— *Male Genitalia* ———

HERNIAS

Early and Late Childhood. Ask the child to try to lift the chair in which you are sitting.

This will help you to detect inguinal and femoral hernias not discovered when the child was asked to cough or strain down.

—*Examination Techniques*—   —*Possible Findings*—

SPECIAL MANEUVER

DETECTION OF PSEUDO-UNDESCENDED TESTICLE. Because the cremasteric reflex is so strong during early and late childhood, examination of the scrotum with the child upright or supine often reveals an undescended testicle. When this occurs, sit the child cross-legged and palpate the inguinal canal and scrotum.

This positioning interrupts the cremasteric reflex and allows the testicle to descend into the scrotum.

The Musculoskeletal System

Screening

Observe the child

- Standing upright with feet together — For foot deformities, bow legs, knock-knees, scoliosis

- Walking and running — For limp and other gait abnormalities due to muscle weakness or spasticity

- Stooping to pick up an object — For eye–hand coordination and muscle balance

—*Examination Techniques*—   —*Possible Findings*—

• Rising from a supine position on the floor	For general neurologic integrity and the proximal leg muscle weakness of muscular dystrophy (**Gower's sign**)

THE SPINE

Inspect and palpate the lumbosacral spine carefully.

• Look and feel for defects of the vertebral bodies.

Defects (spina bifida occulta) may be associated with an underlying spinal cord anomaly (diastematomyelia).

• Look for abnormalities of the skin, pigmented spots, hairy patches, or deep pits that might overlie external openings of sinus tracts that extend to the spinal canal.

A sinus tract provides potential entry to the spinal canal of organisms that can cause meningitis.

SPECIAL MANEUVERS

ORTOLANI TEST. With the infant supine and its legs pointing toward you, flex the legs to 90° at the hips and knees. Place your index fingers over the greater trochanters of the femurs and your thumbs over the lesser trochanters.

When a congenitally dislocated hip is present in a newborn, a click is heard or felt as the femoral head enters the acetabulum near the end of abduction (**Ortolani's sign**). In older infants, decreased abduction of the affected hip(s) may

—*Examination Techniques*—	—*Possible Findings*—
Abduct both hips simultaneously until the lateral aspect of each knee touches the examining table.	be the only finding of dislocation.
TRENDELENBURG TEST. Observe the patient from behind as the weight is shifted from one leg to the other.	
Note if the pelvis remains level (negative sign) or tilts toward the opposite side (positive sign).	A positive Trendelenburg sign is present in diseases of the hip associated with gluteus medius muscle weakness.

——— *The Nervous System* ———

REFLEXES

Infancy. Because the corticospinal pathways are not fully developed at birth, the spinal reflex mechanisms are variable during infancy.

- *Triceps*—Usually not present until after 6 months

- *Abdominals*—Absent at birth, but appear within 6 months

- *Ankle*—Unsustained ankle clonus (8 to 10 beats) is normal.

Sustained ankle clonus suggests severe CNS disease.

—*Examination Techniques*—   —*Possible Findings*—

- *Plantar*—Babinski response present in some (<10%) normal newborns and may remain for as long as 2 years

INFANTILE AUTOMATISMS

Specific reflex activities that test brainstem and spinal cord functions are found in newborns and disappear in early infancy.

Presence or absence of these reflexes does not predict immediate or eventual cortical function positively or negatively. However, absence in the newborn or their persistance beyond their expected time of disappearance suggests severe CNS disease.

PALMAR GRASP REFLEX —disappears at 3 to 4 months

With the baby's head in the midline position and the arms semiflexed, place your index fingers from the ulnar side into the baby's hands and press against the palmar surfaces.

The baby responds by flexing all of its fingers to grasp your fingers.

ROOTING REFLEX—disappears at 3 to 4 months; may be present longer during sleep

With the baby's head in the midline position and hands resting on the anterior chest, stroke with your forefinger the skin at the corners of the mouth.

The mouth opens and the head turns to the stroked side.

—*Examination Techniques*—	—*Possible Findings*—
Stroke the middle of the upper lip.	The mouth opens and the head extends.
Stroke the middle of the lower lip.	The mouth opens and the chin drops.

TRUNK INCURVATION (GALANT'S) REFLEX—disappears at 2 months

| Suspend the baby prone in one of your hands. | |
| Stimulate one side of the baby's back approximately 1 cm from the midline along a paravertebral line extending from the shoulder to the buttocks. | The trunk curves toward the stimulated side with movement of the shoulders and pelvis in that direction. |

VENTRAL SUSPENSION POSITIONING—disappears after 4 months

| Suspend the baby upright facing you with your hands under the arms. | Normally, the head is maintained in the midline and the legs flex at the hips and knees. Fixed extension and crossed adduction of the legs (scissoring) indicate spastic paraplegia or diplegia. |

PLACING RESPONSE—best after 4 days; disappearance time variable

| Hold the baby upright facing away from you with your hands under the arms and your thumbs supporting the back of the head. | The foot is lifted reflexly and placed on the table top. |

—*Examination Techniques*—	—*Possible Findings*—

Allow the dorsal surface of one foot to touch the undersurface of a table top, taking care not to plantar flex the foot. Repeat the process with the other foot.

Once both feet are placed on the table top, propel the baby forward slowly.

A series of alternate stepping movements of the legs and feet occurs.

ROTATION TEST—disappearance time variable

Suspend the baby upright facing you with your hands under the arms. Turn yourself around in one direction and then the other.

The baby's head turns in the direction in which you turn.

Restrain the baby's head with your thumbs as you turn.

The baby's eyes turn in the direction in which you turn.

TONIC NECK REFLEX—may be present at birth, but usually appears at 2 months and disappears at 6 months

With the baby supine, turn its head to one side and hold its chin over its shoulder.

The arm and leg on the side to which the head is turned extend, while the other arm and leg flex. The reflex is considered abnormal when it occurs every time it is evoked.

PEREZ REFLEX—disappears after 3 months

—*Examination Techniques*—	—*Possible Findings*—
Suspend the baby prone in one of your hands. Press the thumb of your other hand over the sacrum and move it firmly over the spine upward to the neck.	The head and spine extend, the knees flex on the abdomen, and the baby cries and urinates.

MORO RESPONSE OR STARTLE REFLEX—disappears by 4 months

Hold the baby in the supine position, supporting the head, back, and legs. Then suddenly lower the entire body about 2 feet and stop abruptly; or—	The arms abduct briskly and extend at the elbows with the hands open and the fingers extended; the legs flex slightly and abduct, but less so than the arms. The arms then come forward over the body in a clasping movement, and simultaneously the baby cries.
Lift the supine baby's head to an angle approximately 30° from the examining table. Suddenly release your grip and allow the head to fall backward, catching it before it hits the table; or—	
Hold the baby supine, supporting the back and pelvis with one hand and arm and the head with the other hand. Then allow the head to drop several centimeters with a sudden, rapid movement; or—	
Produce a loud noise (*e.g.*, strike the examining table with the palms of your hands on both sides of the baby's head).	

4

Aids to Interpretation

Levels of Consciousness

NORMAL
Alert, awake, aware of both self and environment, and responsive to external stimuli

DROWSINESS OR OBTUNDATION
Not fully alert. Consciousness clouded and attentiveness impaired. Thinking slow. Spontaneous movement decreased. Responses to questions and commands, but a tendency to fall asleep afterward

STUPOR
Marked reduction in mental and physical activity. Responses to even painful stimuli reduced or inadequate. Reflex activity present

COMA
Totally unresponsive. Reflexes reduced or absent

Disorders of Speech

APHONIA
A disorder of the volume, quality, or pitch of the voice, *e.g.*, hoarseness or whispered voice

DYSARTHRIA
A disorder of articulation involving the lips, tongue, palate, or pharynx

APHASIA
A disorder of language itself

Height/Weight Table for Adults

Height Without Shoes		Men Aged 25–59	
Feet	Inches	Small Frame	Medium Frame
4	9		
4	10		
4	11		
5	0		
5	1	123–129	126–136
5	2	125–131	128–138
5	3	127–133	130–140
5	4	129–135	132–143
5	5	131–137	134–146
5	6	133–140	137–149
5	7	135–143	140–152
5	8	137–146	143–155
5	9	139–149	146–158
5	10	141–152	149–161
5	11	144–155	152–165
6	0	147–159	155–169
6	1	150–163	159–173
6	2	153–167	162–177
6	3	157–171	166–182

(Weight in Pounds Without Clothes)

Years	Women Aged 25–59 Years		
Large Frame	Small Frame	Medium Frame	Large Frame
	99–108	106–118	115–128
	100–110	108–120	117–131
	101–112	110–123	119–134
	103–115	112–126	122–137
133–145	105–118	115–129	125–140
135–148	108–121	118–132	128–144
137–151	111–124	121–135	131–148
139–155	114–127	124–138	134–152
141–159	117–130	127–141	137–156
144–163	120–133	130–144	140–160
147–167	123–136	133–147	143–164
150–171	126–139	136–150	146–167
153–175	129–142	139–153	149–170
156–179	132–145	142–156	152–173
159–183			
163–187			
167–192			
171–197			
176–202			

(Derived from 1983 Metropolitan Height and Weight Tables: Stat Bull Metrop Life Found 64, No. 1: 6–7, 1983)

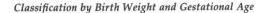

Classification of a Newborn Infant's Level of Maturity

Classification by Birth Weight and Gestational Age

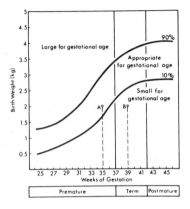

Weight Small for Gestational Age (SGA) = Birth weight < 10th percentile on the intrauterine growth curve

Weight Appropriate for Gestational Age (AGA) = Birth weight within the 10th and 90th percentiles on the intrauterine growth curve

Weight Large for Gestational Age (LGA) = Birth weight > 90th percentile on the intrauterine growth curve

---

Level of intrauterine growth based on birth weight and gestational age of liveborn, single, white infants. Point A represents a premature infant, while point B indicates an infant of similar birth weight who is mature but small for gestational age; the growth curves are representative of the 10th and 90th percentiles for all of the newborns in the sampling.

(Adapted for publication in the Merck Manual 15th edition, 1987, from Sweet AY: Classification of the low-birth-weight infant. In Klaus MH, Fanaroff AA: Care of the High-Risk Neonate, ed 3. Philadelphia, WB Saunders, 1986)

Height and Weight Grids for Girls: Birth to 36 Months

NAME _____ RECORD # _____

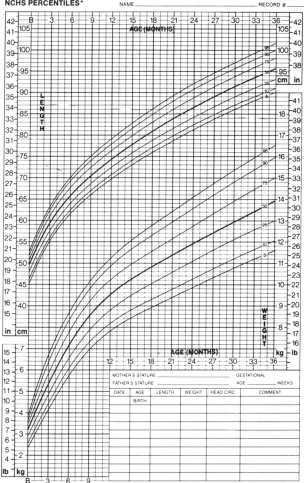

(Adapted from Hamill PVV, Drizd TA, Johnson CL, Reed RB, Roche AF, Moore AM: Physical growth: National Center for Health Statistics percentiles. Am J Clin Nutr 32:607–629, 1979. Data from the National Center for Health Statistics [NCHS], Hyattsville, MD. Figures provided through the courtesy of Ross Laboratories, Columbus, OH)

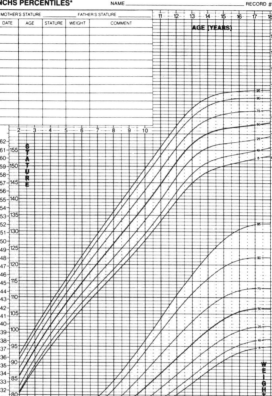

GIRLS: 2 TO 18 YEARS
PHYSICAL GROWTH
NCHS PERCENTILES*

(Adapted from Hamill PVV, Drizd TA, Johnson CL, Reed RB, Roche AF, Moore AM: Physical growth: National Center for Health Statistics percentiles. Am J Clin Nutr 32:607–629, 1979. Data from the National Center for Health Statistics [NCHS], Hyattsville, MD. Figures provided through the courtesy of Ross Laboratories, Columbus, OH)

Height and Weight Grids for Boys: Birth to 36 Months

BOYS: BIRTH TO 36 MONTHS
PHYSICAL GROWTH
NCHS PERCENTILES*

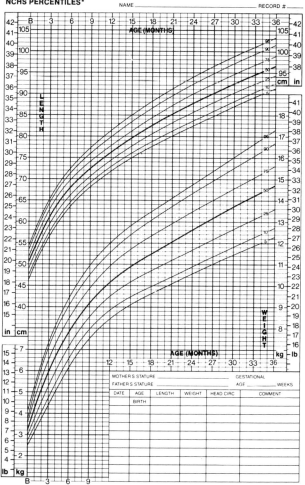

Height and Weight Grids for Boys: 2 to 18 Years

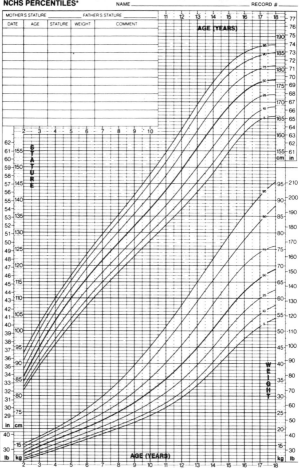

BOYS: 2 TO 18 YEARS
PHYSICAL GROWTH
NCHS PERCENTILES*

(Adapted from Hamill PVV, Drizd TA, Johnson CL, Reed RB, Roche AF, Moore AM: Physical growth: National Center for Health Statistics percentiles. Am J Clin Nutr 32:607–629, 1979. Data from the National Center for Health Statistics [NCHS], Hyattsville, MD. Figures provided through the courtesy of Ross Laboratories, Columbus, OH)

Color Changes in the Skin

Color/Mechanism	Selected Causes
BROWN—increased melanin (greater than a person's genetic norm)	Sun exposure
	Pregnancy (melasma)
	Addison's disease
GRAYISH TAN OR BRONZE—hemosiderin and increased melanin	Hemochromatosis
BLUE (cyanosis)	
Increased deoxyhemoglobin due to hypoxia	
Peripheral	Anxiety or cold environment
Central (arterial)	Heart or lung disease
Abnormal hemoglobin	Methemoglobinemia, sulfhemoglobinemia
RED—increased visibility of oxyhemoglobin due to:	
Dilated superficial blood vessels or increased blood flow in skin	Fever, blushing, alcohol intake, local inflammation
Decreased use of oxygen in skin	Cold exposure (e.g., cold ears)
YELLOW	
Increased bilirubin of jaundice (sclera looks yellow)	Liver disease, hemolysis of red blood cells
Carotenemia (sclera does not look yellow)	Increased carotene intake, anorexia nervosa, some endocrine causes
Retained urinary chromogens, superimposed on the pallor of anemia	Chronic uremia from long-standing kidney disease
PALE	
Decreased melanin	Albinism, vitiligo, tinea versicolor
Decreased visibility of oxyhemoglobin due to:	
Decreased blood flow to skin	Syncope or shock
Decreased amount of oxyhemoglobin	Anemia
Edema (may mask skin pigments)	Nephrotic syndrome

Types of Skin Lesions

Primary Lesions

CIRCUMSCRIBED, FLAT, NONPALPABLE CHANGES IN COLOR

MACULE. Small, up to 1 cm. Examples: freckle, petechia

PATCH. Larger than 1 cm. Example: vitiligo

PALPABLE, ELEVATED, SOLID MASSES

PAPULE. Up to 0.5 cm. Example: the papule of acne

PLAQUE. An elevated flat surface larger than 0.5 cm. Example: xanthelasma of the eyelids

NODULE. 0.5 cm to 1–2 cm; often deeper and firmer than a papule. Example: sebaceous cyst

TUMOR. Larger than 1–2 cm. Example: a large neurofibroma

WHEAL. A relatively transient, superficial area of local skin edema. Example: mosquito bite

CIRCUMSCRIBED SUPERFICIAL ELEVATIONS OF THE SKIN FORMED BY FREE FLUID IN A CAVITY BETWEEN THE SKIN LAYERS

VESICLE. Up to 0.5 cm; filled with serous fluid. Example: poison ivy

BULLA. Greater than 0.5 cm; filled with serous fluid. Example: 2nd-degree burn

PUSTULE. Filled with pus. Example: acne

Secondary Lesions

LOSS OF SKIN SURFACE

EROSION. Loss of superficial epidermis, leaving a moist area that does not bleed. Example: skin surface after a ruptured vesicle

ULCER. A deeper loss of surface that may bleed and scar. Examples: syphilitic chancre, ulcer of venous insufficiency

FISSURE. A linear crack. Example: athlete's foot

MATERIAL ON THE SKIN SURFACE

CRUST. The dried residue of serum, pus, or blood. Example: a scab

SCALE. A thin flake of exfoliated epidermis. Examples: dry skin, dandruff

Visual Fields

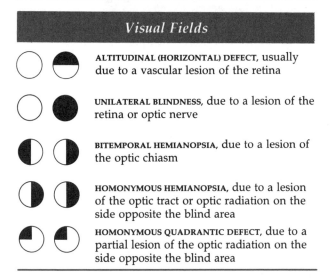

ALTITUDINAL (HORIZONTAL) DEFECT, usually due to a vascular lesion of the retina

UNILATERAL BLINDNESS, due to a lesion of the retina or optic nerve

BITEMPORAL HEMIANOPSIA, due to a lesion of the optic chiasm

HOMONYMOUS HEMIANOPSIA, due to a lesion of the optic tract or optic radiation on the side opposite the blind area

HOMONYMOUS QUADRANTIC DEFECT, due to a partial lesion of the optic radiation on the side opposite the blind area

Physical Findings In and Around the Eye

HERNIATED FAT. A common cause of swelling in the lower lid and the inner third of the upper lid; associated with aging

PERIORBITAL EDEMA. Swelling of the eyelids from excessive fluid; many causes

PTOSIS. A drooping upper eyelid that narrows the palpebral fissure; due to a muscle or nerve disorder

ENLARGED PALPEBRAL FISSURE. Due either to retraction of the eyelids or to exophthalmos, both signs of hyperthyroidism

ECTROPION. Outward turning of the margin of the lower lid, exposing the palpebral conjunctiva

ENTROPION. Inward turning of the lid margin, causing irritation of the cornea or conjunctiva

PINGUECULAE. Harmless yellowish nodules in the bulbar conjunctiva on either side of the iris; associated with aging

XANTHELASMA. Yellowish plaques in the eyelids that may be due to a lipid disorder

BASAL CELL EPITHELIOMA. A common skin cancer

CHALAZION. A beady nodule in either eyelid due to a chronically inflamed meibomian gland

STY. A pimple-like infection around a hair follicle near the lid margin

DACRYOCYSTITIS. An inflammation of the nasolacrimal sac, acute or chronic, that may obstruct tear drainage

CORNEAL ARCUS. A grayish white arc or ring often associated with aging

PTERYGIUM. A thickening of the bulbar conjunctiva that may grow across the cornea

Red Eyes

	Pain	Vision	Ocular Discharge	Pupil	Cornea
CONJUNCTIVITIS	Mild or no discomfort	Only temporary blurring from discharge	Present	Normal	Clear
CILIARY INJECTION					
OF CORNEAL ORIGIN	Present, superficial	Usually decreased	Present	Normal, unless iritis ensues	Varies with cause
ACUTE IRITIS	Present, aching, deep	Decreased	Absent	Small	Clear or slightly clouded
ACUTE GLAUCOMA	Present, aching, deep	Decreased	Absent	Dilated	Steamy, cloudy
SUBCONJUNCTIVAL HEMORRHAGE	Absent	Normal	Absent	Normal	Clear

Pupillary Abnormalities

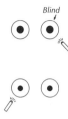

Blind

BLIND EYE. Neither a direct nor a consensual response to light occurs when this blind left eye is stimulated. Normal responses occur when the normal right eye is so stimulated.

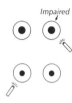

Impaired

MARCUS GUNN (DEAFFERENTED) PUPIL. Diminished direct and consensual responses occur when an eye, impaired by an optic nerve disorder, is stimulated by light. Testing this normal right eye causes normal responses. When the light is swung back to the impaired left eye, the pupils dilate.

HORNER'S SYNDROME. A small pupil due to interruption of its sympathetic nerve supply. Ptosis is associated. Pupillary reactions are normal.

OCULOMOTOR NERVE PARALYSIS. A large pupil, often associated with ptosis of the lid and lateral deviation of the eye. No pupillary reactions in that eye.

TONIC PUPIL. A large pupil with decreased or absent reaction to light and a slow response to near effort

ARGYLL ROBERTSON PUPILS. Small, irregular pupils that react to near effort but not to light.

DILATED FIXED PUPILS. Associated with drug effects or severe brain damage

SMALL FIXED PUPILS. Associated with miotic eye drops, drugs, or brain damage at the level of the pons

Retinal Lesions

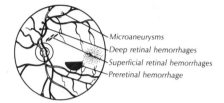

Microaneurysms
Deep retinal hemorrhages
Superficial retinal hemorrhages
Preretinal hemorrhage

RED SPOTS AND STREAKS

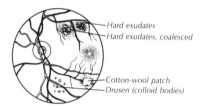

Hard exudates
Hard exudates, coalesced

Cotton-wool patch
Drusen (colloid bodies)

LIGHT-COLORED SPOTS

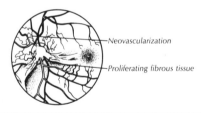

Neovascularization

Proliferating fibrous tissue

CHANGES IN PROLIFERATIVE DIABETIC RETINOPATHY

Abnormal Eardrums

SEROUS EFFUSION

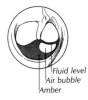

Amber fluid behind the eardrum, with or without air bubbles

Associated with viral upper respiratory infections or sudden changes in atmospheric pressure (diving, flying)

ACUTE OTITIS MEDIA

Red, bulging drum, loss of landmarks

Associated with bacterial infection

TYMPANOSCLEROSIS

A chalky white patch

Scar of an old otitis media; of little or no clinical consequence

PERFORATION

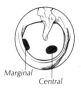

Hole in the eardrum that may be central or marginal

Usually the result of otitis media or trauma

Patterns of Hearing Loss

	Conduction Loss	Sensorineural Loss
IMPAIRED UNDERSTANDING OF WORDS	Minor	Often troublesome
EFFECT OF NOISY ENVIRONMENT	May help	Increases the hearing difficulty
USUAL AGE OF ONSET	Childhood, young adulthood	Middle and old age
EAR CANAL AND DRUM	Often a visible abnormality	The problem not visible
WEBER TEST (IN UNILATERAL HEARING LOSS)	Lateralizes to the impaired ear	Lateralizes to the good ear
RINNE TEST	BC > AC or BC = AC	AC > BC

Abnormalities of the Lips

Chancre   Herpes

HERPES SIMPLEX. Painful vesicles followed by crusting

SYPHILITIC CHANCRE. A firm lesion that ulcerates and may crust

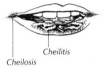

Cheilitis

Cheilosis

ANGULAR STOMATITIS (CHEILOSIS). Softening and cracking at the angles of the mouth

CHEILITIS. Painful cracking, scaling, and crusting of the lower lip

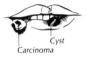

Cyst

Carcinoma

MUCOUS RETENTION CYST. A rounded, soft, often bluish nodule. Benign

CARCINOMA OF THE LIP. A thickened plaque or irregular nodule that may ulcerate or crust. Malignant

PEUTZ-JEGHERS SYNDROME. Brown spots, significant because of their association with intestinal polyposis

ANGIONEUROTIC EDEMA. Diffuse, tense, subcutaneous swelling, usually allergic in cause

Abnormalities of the Gums and Teeth

 GINGIVITIS. Red, swollen gum margins, often due to the formation of calculus on the teeth. *Acute necrotizing gingivitis (Vincent's stomatitis)* is a painful condition that in addition to redness and swelling causes ulceration of the gums and formation of a grayish membrane.

 PERIODONTITIS. A progression of gingivitis to deeper tissues, with resulting recession of the gums and looseness or loss of teeth.

 GINGIVAL ENLARGEMENT. Enlarged gums that partially cover the teeth with heaped-up tissue. A single local enlargement is termed an *epulis.*

 DENTAL CARIES. Tooth decay. Clinically invisible in its early stages, it may produce chalky white spots that later discolor to brown or black, soften, and cavitate.

 HUTCHINSON'S TEETH. A sign of congenital syphilis, most often involving the upper central incisors. These teeth are small, notched, tapered, and widely spaced.

 ABRASION OF TEETH. Irregularities in the biting edges due to recurrent trauma

 ATTRITION OF TEETH. Wear of the teeth. The exposed dentin is often yellow or brown.

Tongues

SMOOTH TONGUE. Due to loss of papillae caused by vitamin B or iron deficiency or possibly anticancer drugs

HAIRY TONGUE. Due to elongated papillae that may look yellowish, brown, or black. Harmless

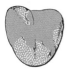
GEOGRAPHIC TONGUE. Scattered areas in which the papillae are lost, giving a map-like appearance. Harmless

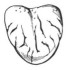
FISSURED TONGUE. Fissures may appear with aging. Harmless

HYPOGLOSSAL NERVE PARALYSIS. Atrophy and fasciculations on the involved side, with deviation of the tongue toward it

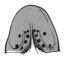
VARICOSE VEINS (CAVIAR LESIONS). Dark round spots on the undersurface of the tongue, associated with aging

CARCINOMA OF THE TONGUE. A malignancy that should be considered in any nodule or nonhealing ulcer at the base or edges of the tongue

Abnormalities of the Pharynx

Swollen, red

Exudate

EXUDATIVE PHARYNGITIS. Associated with streptococcal pharyngitis and some viral illnesses, including infectious mononucleosis. In diphtheria, unlike streptococcal infections, the exudate may spread as a gray membrane over the soft palate and uvula.

PERITONSILLAR ABSCESS. A unilateral, red bulge in the pharynx that may displace the uvula toward the opposite side

UNILATERAL PARALYSIS OF THE VAGUS NERVE. With "ah," the soft palate fails to rise on the involved side and the uvula deviates to the opposite side.

Abnormalities of the Thyroid Gland

DIFFUSE ENLARGEMENT. May be due to Graves' disease, Hashimoto's thyroiditis, endemic goiter (iodine deficiency), or sporadic goiter

MULTINODULAR GOITER. An enlargement with two or more identifiable nodules, usually metabolic in cause

SINGLE NODULE. May be due to a cyst, a benign tumor, or cancer of the thyroid, or may be one palpable nodule in a clinically unrecognized multinodular goiter

Rate and Rhythm of Breathing

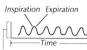

Inspiration Expiration

Time

Volume of air

NORMAL. In adults, 14 to 20 per min; in infants, up to 44 per min

RAPID SHALLOW BREATHING (TACHYPNEA). Many causes, including restrictive lung disease and pleural pain

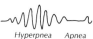

RAPID DEEP BREATHING (HYPERPNEA, HYPERVENTILATION). Many causes, including exercise, anxiety, metabolic acidosis, brainstem injury

SLOW BREATHING. May be due to diabetic coma, drug-induced respiratory depression, increased intracranial pressure

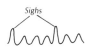

Hyperpnea   Apnea

CHEYNE-STOKES BREATHING. Rhythmically alternating periods of hyperpnea and apnea. In infants and the aged, may be normal during sleep; also accompanies brain damage, heart failure, uremia, and respiratory depression

ATAXIC (BIOT'S) BREATHING. Unpredictable irregularity of depth and rate. Causes include brain damage and respiratory depression.

Sighs

SIGHING RESPIRATION. Breathing punctuated by frequent sighs. When associated with other symptoms, it suggests the hyperventilation syndrome. Occasional sighs are normal.

Lung Lobes

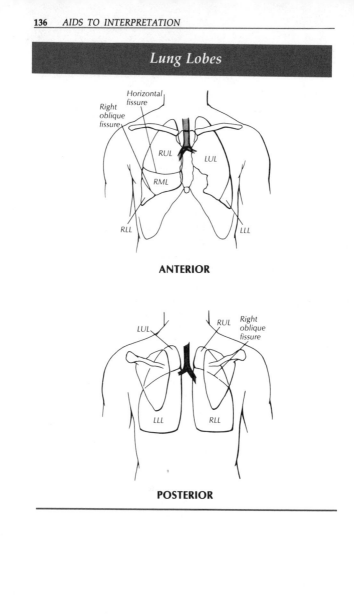

ANTERIOR

POSTERIOR

Deformities of the Thorax

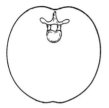

BARREL CHEST. An anteroposterior diameter increased from the adult norm so that the chest (in cross-section) becomes rounded. May accompany aging and chronic obstructive pulmonary disease. (The chest of a normal infant also has this shape.)

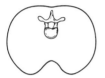

FUNNEL CHEST (PECTUS EXCAVATUM). Posterior displacement of the lower sternum. Compression of the heart or great vessels may cause murmurs.

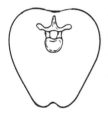

PIGEON CHEST (PECTUS CARINATUM). Anterior displacement of the sternum. The costal cartilages adjacent to the sternum are relatively depressed.

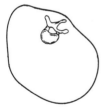

THORACIC KYPHOSCOLIOSIS. A structural spinal curvature associated with distortion and asymmetry of the chest.

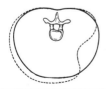

FLAIL CHEST. Abnormal respiratory movements associated with multiple rib fractures. The injured area moves inward in inspiration, outward in expiration.

Percussion Notes

	Relative Intensity, Pitch, and Duration	Examples
FLATNESS	Soft/high/short	Large pleural effusion
DULLNESS	Medium/medium/medium	Lobar pneumonia
RESONANCE	Loud/low/long	Normal lung, bronchitis
HYPERRESONANCE	Louder, lower, longer	Emphysema, pneumothorax
TYMPANY	Loud/high*/*	Large pneumothorax

* Distinguished mainly by musical timbre

Breath Sounds

	Duration	Intensity and Pitch of Expiratory Sound	Example Locations
VESICULAR	Insp > exp	Soft/Low	Most of the lungs
BRONCHO-VESICULAR	Insp = exp	Medium/Medium	1st and 2nd interspaces, interscapular area
BRONCHIAL	Exp > insp	Loud/High	Over the manubrium; lobar pneumonia
TRACHEAL	Insp = exp	Very loud/High	Over the trachea

In the figures above, duration is indicated by the length of the line, intensity by the width of the line, and pitch by the slope of the line.

Transmitted Voice Sounds*

BRONCHOPHONY. Increased loudness and clarity of the spoken voice

EGOPHONY (E-TO-A CHANGE). The spoken "ee" sounds like "ay."

WHISPERED PECTORILOQUY. Increased loudness and clarity of the whispered voice

---

* As heard through the chest wall with a stethoscope

Adventitious Lung Sounds

DISCONTINUOUS SOUNDS (CRACKLES). Intermittent, nonmusical, short sounds, like dots in time

- *Fine crackles* (· · · ·)—soft, high-pitched, very brief
- *Coarse crackles* (• • • •)—somewhat louder, lower-pitched, not quite so brief

CRACKLES CLASSIFIED BY TIMING

- *Late inspiratory crackles.* Must continue into late inspiration. Usually fine, profuse, and heard in dependent portions of the lungs. Causes include interstitial lung disease and early congestive heart failure.
- *Early inspiratory crackles.* Do not continue into late inspiration. Often coarse. Causes include chronic bronchitis and asthma.

CONTINUOUS SOUNDS. Musical and notably longer than crackles, like dashes in time, but not necessarily truly continuous. May be generalized (as in asthma or chronic obstructive lung disease) or persistent and local (as from a tumor or foreign body that is obstructing a bronchus). Clearing by cough or deep breathing suggests secretions as the cause.

- *Wheezes* (〰〰〰)—relatively high-pitched (around 400 Hz or more) with a hissing or shrill quality
- *Rhonchi* (〰〰〰)—relatively low-pitched (around 200 Hz or less) with a snoring quality

STRIDOR. A wheeze heard only or chiefly in inspiration and usually louder in the neck than over the chest. Indicates partial airway obstruction in the neck

PLEURAL RUB. A creaking, grating sound associated with respiratory movements. Originates in inflamed pleural surfaces

Signs in Selected

	Trachea	*Percussion Note*
CHRONIC BRONCHITIS	Midline	Resonant
LEFT HEART FAILURE (EARLY)	Midline	Resonant
LOBAR PNEUMONIA	Midline	Dull
ATELECTASIS (LOBAR)	May be shifted toward	Dull
PLEURAL EFFUSION (LARGE)	May be shifted away	Dull
PNEUMOTHORAX	May be shifted away	Hyperresonant or tympanitic
EMPHYSEMA	Midline	Hyperresonant
BRONCHIAL ASTHMA	Midline	Normal to hyperresonant

Chest Disorders

Breath Sounds	Transmitted Voice Sounds	Adventitious Sounds
Normal	Normal	None, or wheezes, rhonchi, crackles
Normal	Normal	Late inspiratory crackles in lower lungs; possible wheezes
Bronchial	Increased*	Late inspiratory crackles
Usually absent	Usually absent	None
Decreased to absent	Decreased to absent	Usually none; possible pleural rub
Decreased to absent	Decreased to absent	None
Decreased to absent	Decreased to absent	None unless bronchitis also
May be obscured by wheezes	Normal or decreased	Wheezes, perhaps crackles

* With increased tactile fremitus, bronchophony, egophony, whispered pectoriloquy

Sex Maturity Ratings in Girls: Breasts

Stage 1

Preadolescent—elevation of nipple only

Stage 2	Stage 3
Breast bud stage. Elevation of breast and nipple as a small mound; enlargement of areolar diameter	Further enlargement and elevation of breast and areola, with no separation of their contours

Stage 4	Stage 5
Projection of areola and nipple to form a secondary mound above the level of the breast	Mature stage; projection of nipple only. Areola has receded to general contour of the breast (although in some normal individuals the areola continues to form a secondary mound).

Illustrations through the courtesy of W.A. Daniel, Jr.

Sex Maturity Ratings in Girls: Pubic Hair

Stage 1   Preadolescent—no pubic hair except for the fine body hair (vellus hair) similar to that on the abdomen

Stage 2

Stage 3

Sparse growth of long, slightly pigmented, downy hair, straight or only slightly curled, chiefly along the labia

Darker, coarser, curlier hair, spreading sparsely over the pubic symphysis

Stage 4

Stage 5

Coarse and curly hair as in adults; area covered greater than in stage 3 but not as great as in the adult and not yet including the thighs

Hair adult in quantity and quality, spread on the medial surfaces of the thighs but not up over the abdomen

Illustrations through the courtesy of W. A. Daniel, Jr.

Common Breast Nodules

	Gross Cyst	Fibroadenoma	Cancer
USUAL AGE	30–60 years	Puberty and young adulthood, up to age 55	30–90 years
NUMBER	Single or multiple	Usually single, may be multiple	Usually single; other nodules may coexist
SHAPE	Round	Round, discoid, lobular	Irregular or stellate
CONSISTENCY	Soft to firm, usually elastic	May be soft, usually firm	Firm or hard
DELIMITATION	Well circumscribed	Well circumscribed	Not clearly delineated from surrounding tissues
MOBILITY	Mobile	Very mobile	May be fixed
TENDERNESS	Often tender	Usually nontender	Usually nontender
RETRACTION SIGNS	Absent	Absent	May be present

Heart Rates and Rhythms

REGULAR RHYTHMS

FAST (OVER 100)

Sinus tachycardia

Atrial or nodal (supraventricular) tachycardia

Atrial flutter with a regular ventricular response

Ventricular tachycardia

NORMAL (60–100)

Normal sinus rhythm

Atrial flutter with a regular ventricular response

SLOW

Sinus bradycardia

Second-degree heart block

Complete heart block

IRREGULAR RHYTHMS

RHYTHMICALLY OR SPORADICALLY IRREGULAR

Premature contractions (atrial, nodal, or ventricular)

Sinus arrhythmia

TOTALLY IRREGULAR

Atrial fibrillation

Atrial flutter with varying block

	Average Heart Rate of Infants and Children at Rest	
Age	*Average Rate*	*Two Standard Deviations*
Birth	140	50
1st 6 months	130	50
6–12 months	115	40
1–2 years	110	40
2–6 years	103	35
6–10 years	95	30
10–14 years	85	30

RECOMMENDED SIZE OF THE INFLATABLE BAG

Width 75% of the upper arm or upper leg length

Length 100% or more of the upper arm or upper leg circumference

METHOD

Same as for adults in children 3 years and older

Use flush method for infants and younger children (see Chapter 3, p. 94).

CLASSIFICATION OF BLOOD PRESSURE LEVELS IN CHILDREN

NORMAL: Systolic and diastolic BPs < 90th percentile for age and sex

HIGH NORMAL: Average systolic and diastolic BPs between the 90th and 95th percentiles for age and sex

HIGH (HYPERTENSION): Average systolic and/or diastolic BPs ≥ 95th percentile for age and sex

AGE-SPECIFIC PERCENTILES OF BLOOD PRESSURE MEASUREMENTS IN CHILDREN

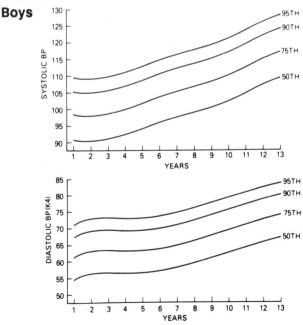

Boys

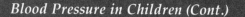

Blood Pressure in Children (Cont.)

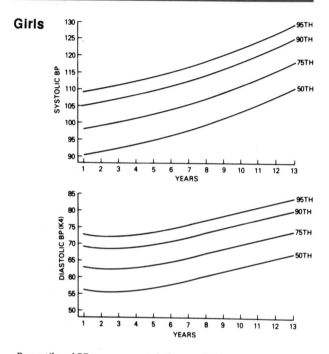

Percentiles of BP measurements in boys and girls 1 to 13 years of age. K4 = Korotkoff phase-IV sound (low-pitched and muffled).

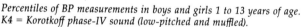

(Reproduced with permission from the Second Task Force on Blood Pressure Control in Children of the National Heart, Lung, and Blood Institute. Pediatrics [Suppl] 79:1–25, 1987)

Blood Pressure

RECOMMENDED SIZE OF THE INFLATABLE BAG

Width 40% of the arm circumference

Length 80% of the arm circumference

DIASTOLIC PRESSURE: The disappearance point of Korotkoff sounds in adults, the muffle point in children

METHODS OF INTENSIFYING KOROTKOFF SOUNDS

1. Raise the patient's arm before and during inflation, then lower the arm and take the blood pressure.
2. Inflate the cuff, ask the patient to make a fist several times, and take the blood pressure.

CLASSIFICATION OF BLOOD PRESSURE LEVELS IN ADULTS

Confirm by two or more measurements on each of three separate visits.

DIASTOLIC LEVEL (in mm Hg)

Severe hypertension	≥115
Moderate hypertension	105–114
Mild hypertension	90–104
High normal BP	85–89

SYSTOLIC LEVEL when diastolic pressure is <90

Isolated systolic hypertension	≥160
Borderline isolated systolic hypertension	140–159

NORMAL BLOOD PRESSURE: Diastolic <85, systolic <140

ORTHOSTATIC (POSTURAL) HYPOTENSION: A decrease of 15 mm Hg or more in systolic pressure or any decrease in diastolic pressure when the patient changes from the supine to a sitting or standing position

The Apical Impulse

	Normal	Hyperkinetic	Pressure Overload	Volume Overload
LOCATION	5th or 4th left interspace, inside midclavicular line	Normal	Normal	Displaced to the left and possibly downward
DIAMETER	Little more than 2 cm (1 cm in children); ≤3 cm when patient lies on left side	Normal	Increased	Increased
AMPLITUDE	Small, gentle	Increased	Increased	Increased
DURATION	Less than ⅔ of systole, stops before S_2	Normal	Prolonged, perhaps up to S_2	Often slightly prolonged
EXAMPLES OF CAUSES		Anxiety, hyperthyroidism, severe anemia	Hypertension, aortic stenosis	Aortic or mitral regurgitation

Heart Sounds

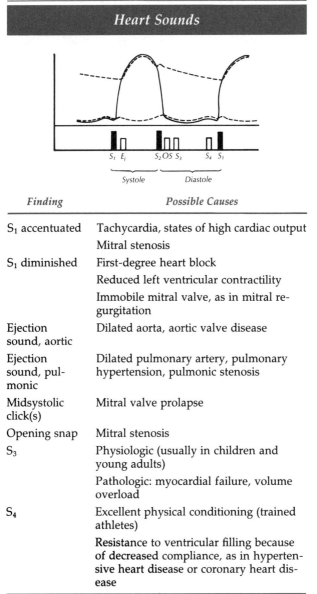

Finding	Possible Causes
S_1 accentuated	Tachycardia, states of high cardiac output
	Mitral stenosis
S_1 diminished	First-degree heart block
	Reduced left ventricular contractility
	Immobile mitral valve, as in mitral regurgitation
Ejection sound, aortic	Dilated aorta, aortic valve disease
Ejection sound, pulmonic	Dilated pulmonary artery, pulmonary hypertension, pulmonic stenosis
Midsystolic click(s)	Mitral valve prolapse
Opening snap	Mitral stenosis
S_3	Physiologic (usually in children and young adults)
	Pathologic: myocardial failure, volume overload
S_4	Excellent physical conditioning (trained athletes)
	Resistance to ventricular filling because of decreased compliance, as in hypertensive heart disease or coronary heart disease

An Apparently Split First Heart Sound

	Left-Sided S_4	Split S_1	Aortic Ejection Sound	Early Systolic Click
	‖ │	│ᵢ │	‖ │	‖ │
BEST HEARD AT	Apex	Lower left sternal border	Right 2nd interspace, apex, or both	At or medial to apex or at left sternal border
PITCH	Low	High	High	High
QUALITY	Dull	Both components similar	Clicking	Clicking
LOUDER WITH	Bell	Diaphragm	Diaphragm	Diaphragm
PALPABLE SPLIT	May be present	Absent	Absent	Absent
AIDS	Partial left lateral decubitus position	None	None	Click delayed by squatting

Heart Murmurs and Similar Sounds

Likely Causes

MIDSYSTOLIC

Innocent murmurs (no cardiovascular abnormality)

Physiologic murmurs (from increased flow across a semilunar valve, as in pregnancy, fever, anemia)

Aortic stenosis

Murmurs that mimic aortic stenosis (aortic sclerosis, bicuspid aortic valve, dilated aorta, and pathologically increased systolic flow across the aortic valve)

Hypertrophic cardiomyopathy

Pulmonic stenosis

PANSYSTOLIC

Mitral regurgitation

Tricuspid regurgitation

Ventricular septal defect

LATE SYSTOLIC

Mitral valve prolapse

EARLY DIASTOLIC

Aortic regurgitation

MID-DIASTOLIC AND PRESYSTOLIC

Mitral stenosis

CONTINUOUS MURMURS AND MURMUR-LIKE SOUNDS

Patent ductus arteriosus

Pericardial friction rub (a scratchy sound with 1–3 components)

Venous hum

Cyanosis and Congenital Heart Disease

No Cyanosis	Early Cyanosis	Late Cyanosis
Small septal defects		Large septal defects
Mild pure pulmonic stenosis	Severe pulmonic stenosis with intact ventricular system	Mild pure pulmonic stenosis
Coarctation of the aorta	Severe tetralogy of Fallot	Less severe tetralogy of Fallot
Patent ductus arteriosus	Tricuspid atresia	Eisenmenger complex
Anomalous origin of left coronary artery	Two- and three-chambered hearts	
Subendocardial fibroelastosis	Transposition of the great vessels	
Glycogen storage disease		

Tender Abdomens

Visceral Tenderness   *Peritoneal Tenderness*

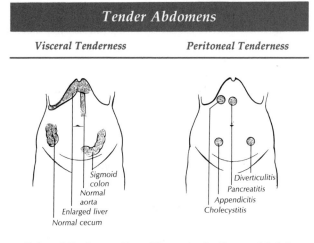

Sigmoid
colon
Normal
aorta
Enlarged liver
Normal cecum

Diverticulitis
Pancreatitis
Appendicitis
Cholecystitis

Referred Tenderness From Disease in the Chest and Pelvis

Acute Pleurisy   *Acute Salpingitis*

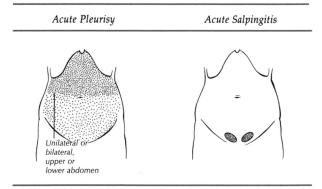

Unilateral or
bilateral,
upper or
lower abdomen

Sex Maturity Ratings in Boys

In assigning SMRs in boys, observe each of the three characteristics separately. Record two separate ratings: pubic hair and genital. If the penis and testes differ in their stages, average the two into a single figure for the genital rating.

		Pubic Hair
Stage 1		Predolescent—no pubic hair except for the fine body hair (vellus hair) similar to that on the abdomen
Stage 2		Sparse growth of long, slightly pigmented, downy hair, straight or only slightly curled, chiefly at the base of the penis
Stage 3		Darker, coarser, curlier hair spreading sparsely over the pubic symphysis
Stage 4		Coarse and curly hair, as in the adult; area covered greater than in stage 3 but not as great as in the adult and not yet including the thighs
Stage 5		Hair adult in quantity and quality, spread to the medial surfaces of the thighs but not up over the abdomen

Sex Maturity Ratings in Boys (Cont.)

	Genital	
Penis		*Testes and Scrotum*
Preadolescent—same size and proportions as in childhood		Preadolescent—same size and proportions as in childhood
Slight or no enlargement		Testes larger; scrotum larger, somewhat reddened, and altered in texture
Larger, especially in length		Further enlarged
Further enlarged in length and breadth, with development of the glans		Further enlarged; scrotal skin darkened
Adult in size and shape		Adult in size and shape

Illustrations through the courtesy of W.A. Daniel, Jr.

Abnormalities in the Scrotum

SCROTAL HERNIA. Protrusion of abdominal contents through the external inguinal ring into the scrotum. The clinician's fingers cannot get above the mass.

HYDROCELE. A fluid-filled sac in the tunica vaginalis. The clinician's fingers can get above the scrotal mass.

ACUTE ORCHITIS. An acutely tender, swollen testis due to infection

ACUTE EPIDIDYMITIS. A tender, swollen epididymis, usually associated with infection of the urinary tract or prostate

TUBERCULOUS EPIDIDYMITIS. Chronic inflammatory enlargement of the epididymis, often with thickening of the vas deferens

VARICOCELE. Varicose veins of the spermatic cord, traditionally described as feeling like a "bag of worms"

TUMOR OF THE TESTIS. A usually painless solid nodule or mass in the testis

 CYST OF THE EPIDIDYMIS. A small, painless, fluid-filled mass above the testis. A *spermatocele* is clinically like a cyst but contains sperm.

 TORSION OF THE SPERMATIC CORD. An acutely tender, swollen testis due to twisting of the organ on the spermatic cord, with resulting circulatory impairment

 SMALL TESTIS. Small firm testes suggestive of Klinefelter's syndrome; small soft testis(es) suggestive of atrophy

CRYPTORCHIDISM. An undescended testicle, not palpable in the scrotum. The scrotal sac is poorly developed on the involved side(s).

Abnormalities of the Penis

HYPOSPADIAS. Congenital displacement of the urethral meatus to the inferior surface of the penis

PHIMOSIS. A tight prepuce that cannot be retracted

PARAPHIMOSIS. A tight prepuce that, once retracted, cannot be replaced over the glans

BALANITIS. Inflammation of the glans

BALANOPOSTHITIS. Inflammation of the glans and prepuce.

CHANCRE. A usually nontender, firm erosion or ulcer, typically on the glans; due to primary syphilis

GENITAL HERPES. A cluster of small vesicles, typically on the glans, that evolve into painful small ulcers on red bases

VENEREAL WARTS. Warty growths on the glans, shaft, or base of the penis; due to human papillomavirus

CANCER OF THE PENIS. An indurated and usually nontender nodule or ulcer of the glans or inner surface of the prepuce. Seen mainly in uncircumcised men

Abnormalities on Rectal Examination

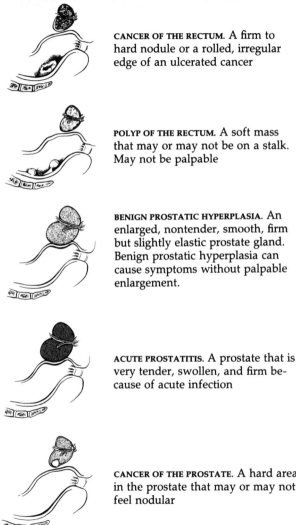

CANCER OF THE RECTUM. A firm to hard nodule or a rolled, irregular edge of an ulcerated cancer

POLYP OF THE RECTUM. A soft mass that may or may not be on a stalk. May not be palpable

BENIGN PROSTATIC HYPERPLASIA. An enlarged, nontender, smooth, firm but slightly elastic prostate gland. Benign prostatic hyperplasia can cause symptoms without palpable enlargement.

ACUTE PROSTATITIS. A prostate that is very tender, swollen, and firm because of acute infection

CANCER OF THE PROSTATE. A hard area in the prostate that may or may not feel nodular

Abnormalities of the Vulva and Urethral Meatus

ULCERS OF THE VULVA

SYPHILITIC CHANCRE. Usually firm and painless, often but not necessarily single

GENITAL HERPES. Painful, shallow, on red bases; usually several or multiple

ULCERATED CARCINOMA OF THE VULVA. Most common in elderly women but not limited exclusively to them

RAISED LESIONS ON THE VULVA

SEBACEOUS (INCLUSION) CYST. Small, firm, round, smooth

VENEREAL WARTS (CONDYLOMATA ACUMINATA). Irregular in surface (warty), often multiple

SECONDARY SYPHILIS (CONDYLOMATA LATA). Slightly raised, flattened papules, round or oval, covered by a gray exudate

CARCINOMA OF THE VULVA. Raised, red, variable in appearance, may be ulcerated

BARTHOLIN'S GLAND INFECTION. A swelling in the posterior labium; tender and red when acute, cystic when chronic

RED SWELLINGS OF THE URETHRAL MEATUS

URETHRAL CARUNCLE. A small swelling on the posterior aspect of the urethral meatus

PROLAPSED URETHRAL MUCOSA. A ring of swollen red mucosa surrounding the urethral meatus

Relaxations of the Pelvic Floor

When the pelvic floor is weakened, various structures may become displaced. These displacements are seen best when the patient strains down.

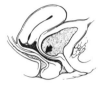

A CYSTOCELE is a bulge of the anterior wall of the upper part of the vagina, together with the urinary bladder above it.

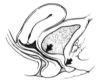

A CYSTOURETHROCELE involves both the bladder and the urethra as they bulge into the anterior vaginal wall throughout most of its extent.

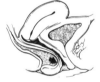

A RECTOCELE is a bulge of the posterior vaginal wall, together with a portion of the rectum.

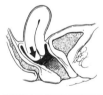

A PROLAPSED UTERUS has descended down the vaginal canal. There are three degrees of severity: first, still within the vagina (as illustrated); second, with the cervix at the introitus; and third, with the cervix outside the introitus.

Vaginitis

	Discharge	Symptoms and Signs
TRICHOMONAS VAGINITIS	Yellowish green, often profuse, may be malodorous	Itching, dysuria, dyspareunia Vulva sometimes red Vagina may be diffusely red with granular red spots or petechiae.
CANDIDA (MONILIA) VAGINITIS	White, curdy, often thick, not malodorous	Itching, vaginal soreness, external dysuria, dyspareunia Vulva often red and swollen Vagina often red with white patches of discharge
BACTERIAL VAGINOSIS	Gray or white, thin, homogeneous, malodorous; seldom profuse	Fishy genital odor Vulva and vaginal mucosa usually look normal.
ATROPHIC VAGINITIS	Variable in color, consistency, and amount; may be blood-tinged; rarely profuse	Itching, vaginal soreness, dyspareunia Vulva atrophic Vaginal mucosa dry, pale; may be red, petechial, or ecchymotic; possible erosions or adhesions

Common Variations in the Cervix

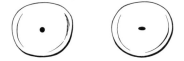

THE OS may be round, oval, or slitlike.

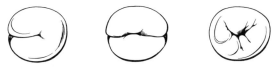

LACERATIONS from vaginal deliveries may be unilateral transverse, bilateral transverse, or stellate.

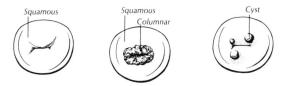

Squamous   *Squamous*   *Cyst*
Columnar

THE EPITHELIUM of a normal cervix may be all squamous or both squamous and columnar. Nabothian cysts may be present.

Abnormalities of the Cervix

CARCINOMA OF THE CERVIX. An irregular, hard mass suggests cancer. Early lesions cannot be detected by physical examination alone.

ENDOCERVICAL POLYP. A bright red, smooth mass that protrudes from the os suggests a polyp. It bleeds easily.

MUCOPURULENT CERVICITIS. A yellowish exudate emerging from the cervical os suggests this diagnosis. Causes include *Chlamydia* and gonococcal infections.

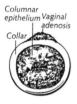

Columnar epithelium
Vaginal adenosis
Collar

FETAL EXPOSURE TO DIETHYLSTILBESTROL. Several changes may be seen: a collar of tissue around the cervix, columnar epithelium that covers the cervix or extends to the vaginal wall (then termed vaginal adenosis), and, rarely, carcinoma of the vagina.

Positions of the Uterus and Uterine Myomas

 AN ANTEVERTED UTERUS lies in a forward position at roughly a right angle to the vagina. This is the most common position. **Anteflexion**—a forward flexion of the uterine body in relation to the cervix—often coexists.

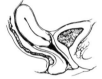 **A RETROVERTED UTERUS** is tilted posteriorly with its cervix facing anteriorly.

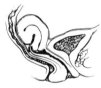 **A RETROFLEXED UTERUS** has a posterior tilt that involves the uterine body but not the cervix. A uterus that is retroflexed or retroverted may be felt only through the rectal wall; some cannot be felt at all.

 A MYOMA OF THE UTERUS is a very common, benign tumor that feels firm and often irregular. There may be more than one. A myoma on the posterior surface of the uterus may be mistaken for a retrodisplaced uterus; one on the anterior surface may be mistaken for an anteverted uterus.

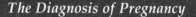

The Diagnosis of Pregnancy

In weeks or months from the last menstrual period

6TH WEEK*

Softening of the uterine isthmus—the first clinical manifestation of pregnancy (**Hegar's sign**)

Rounding of the fundus into a globular shape that may become asymmetrical at the site of fetal implantation

2ND MONTH

Softening at the cervix so that it feels like lips, not like the nose

Purplish color of the vaginal and cervical mucosa

12TH THROUGH 36TH WEEK

A rise in the fundal height:

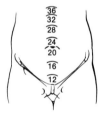

Chronic Vascular Insufficiency

	Arterial	*Deep Venous*
PAIN	Intermittent claudication, possibly pain at rest	Aching on dependency
PULSES	Decreased or absent	Normal, but may be obscured by edema
COLOR	Pallor on elevation, rubor on dependency	Normal, or cyanotic on dependency. Pigmentation around the ankle
TEMPERATURE	Cool	Normal
EDEMA	Absent or mild	Present, often marked
SKIN CHANGES	Thin, shiny, atrophic; decreased hair; ridged, thickened nails	Brown pigment near the ankle, stasis dermatitis, and possible thickening of the skin with narrowing of the leg
ULCERS, IF ANY	Toes, points of trauma	At the sides of the ankle, especially medially
GANGRENE	May be present	Absent

Peripheral Causes of Edema

	Orthostatic Edema	Lymph-edema	Lipedema	Deep Venous Insufficiency
EDEMA	Soft, pitting	Soft early, becomes hard and nonpitting	Minimal, if any	Soft, pitting; may become hard and nonpitting
SKIN THICKENING	Absent	Marked	Absent	Occasional
ULCERATION	Absent	Rare	Absent	Common
PIGMENTATION	Absent	Absent	Absent	Common
FOOT SWELLING	Yes	Yes	No	Yes
BILATERALITY	Always	Often	Always	Occasional

Abnormalities of the Hands

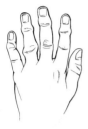

OSTEOARTHRITIS. Hard, dorsolateral nodules on the distal interphalangeal joints (Heberden's nodes) and, less commonly, similar nodules on the proximal interphalangeal joints (Bouchard's nodes)

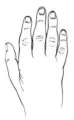

ACUTE RHEUMATOID ARTHRITIS. Tenderness, pain, stiffness, and swelling, affecting mainly the proximal interphalangeal and metacarpophalangeal joints.

CHRONIC RHEUMATOID ARTHRITIS. Chronic swelling and thickening of the proximal interphalangeal and metacarpophalangeal joints; ulnar deviation of the fingers; muscular atrophy; rheumatoid nodules

Boutonniere (A) and swan neck (B) deformities may also be seen.

(Table continued on next page)

Abnormalities of the Hands (Cont.)

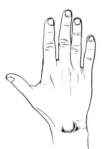

GANGLION. A cystic, round, usually nontender swelling along a tendon sheath or joint capsule. The wrist is a common site, but a ganglion may occur elsewhere.

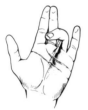

DUPUYTREN'S CONTRACTURE. A thickening of the palmar fascia, first felt as a nodule near the distal palmar crease. A fibrotic cord then develops, and a flexion contraction involving the finger may ensue.

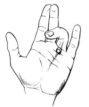

TRIGGER FINGER. A painless nodule in a flexor tendon of the palm, near the head of the metacarpal. Too big to slide easily into the tendon sheath on extension, it necessitates extra effort or force. A snap is felt and heard when it pops through.

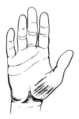

THENAR ATROPHY. Wasting of the muscles of the thenar eminence. It suggests a disorder of the median nerve.

Swollen or Tender Elbows

Lateral
epicondylitis

Arthritis

Olecranon bursitis

Rheumatoid
nodules

EPICONDYLITIS A painful, tender lateral epicondyle suggests *lateral epicondylitis* (tennis elbow). Extension of the elbow against resistance increases the pain.

A painful, tender medial epicondyle (not illustrated) suggests *medial epicondylitis* (pitcher's or Little League elbow). Wrist flexion against resistance increases the pain.

ARTHRITIS Tenderness and swelling in the groove between the olecranon process and the lateral epicondyle suggest arthritis of the elbow joint.

OLECRANON BURSITIS Swelling superficial to the olecranon bursa suggests olecranon bursitis. It may be acute or chronic.

RHEUMATOID NODULES Rheumatoid nodules are subcutaneous, firm, and nontender. They occur along the extensor surface of the ulna and may or may not be attached to the underlying periosteum. They are associated with rheumatoid arthritis.

Painful, Tender Shoulders

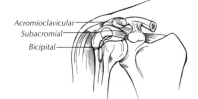

Acromioclavicular
Subacromial
Bicipital

SUBACROMIAL TENDERNESS	Tenderness in the subacromial area suggests either *rotator cuff tendinitis* (the impingement syndrome) or *calcific tendinitis*. The latter typically has a more acute onset and course.
TENDERNESS OVER THE BICEPS TENDON	Tenderness over the long head of the biceps tendon suggests *bicipital tendinitis*. With the patient's arm at the side and the elbow flexed to 90°, supination against resistance increases the pain.
ACROMIO-CLAVICULAR JOINT TENDER-NESS	Tenderness over the acromioclavicular joint (in the absence of recent injury that could also explain it) suggests acromioclavicular arthritis. Shrugging the shoulders often increases the pain but movement limited to the glenohumeral joint does not.

Abnormalities of the Feet

ACUTE GOUTY ARTHRITIS. A hot, red, painful, and tender swelling often involving the first metatarsophalangeal joint

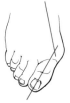

HALLUX VALGUS. A lateral deviation of the great toe. The first metatarsal may be deviated medially. A bursa may form between the joint and the skin and become inflamed (a bunion).

HAMMER TOE. Hyperextension at the metatarsophalangeal joint with flexion at the proximal interphalangeal joint

PLANTAR WART. A wart in the thick skin of the sole. It may be covered by a callus. Look for the small dark spots of a wart.

NEUROTROPHIC ULCER. A painless, often deep ulcer typically surrounded by callus. It occurs at pressure points in patients whose pain sensation is decreased or absent.

CLUBFOOT (TALIPES EQUINOVARUS DEFORMITY). Characterized by forefoot adduction, and inversion and plantar flexion (equinus position) of the entire foot

Spinal Curvatures

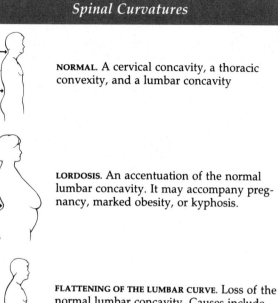

NORMAL. A cervical concavity, a thoracic convexity, and a lumbar concavity

LORDOSIS. An accentuation of the normal lumbar concavity. It may accompany pregnancy, marked obesity, or kyphosis.

FLATTENING OF THE LUMBAR CURVE. Loss of the normal lumbar concavity. Causes include muscle spasm and ankylosing spondylitis.

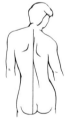

LIST. A lateral tilt of the spine. A plumb line dropped from T1 falls lateral to the gluteal cleft. Muscle spasm associated with a herniated disc is a common cause.

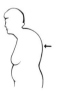

KYPHOSIS. An exaggerated, rounded thoracic convexity. It is common in aging, especially in women.

GIBBUS. An angular, localized convexity due to one or more collapsed vertebrae. Causes include metastatic cancer and tuberculosis of the spine.

SCOLIOSIS. A lateral curvature of the spine. It is described by the location and direction of its chief convexity, here a thoracic scoliosis with convexity to the right. Compensating curves usually correct any list. Forward flexion often makes the deformity more evident.

Gait and Posture

SPASTIC HEMIPARESIS. Arm held close to the side with joints flexed. Leg extended and ankle plantar flexed. On walking, the toe scrapes or the leg is circumducted.

SCISSORS GAIT (BILATERAL SPASTIC PARESIS). A stiff gait in which the thighs cross forward on each other with each step

STEPPAGE GAIT (LOWER MOTOR NEURON WEAKNESS). Because of foot drop, either dragging of the feet or lifting them high and slapping them down

SENSORY ATAXIA. Unsteady, wide-based gait, partially corrected by watching the ground. Romberg test is positive.

CEREBELLAR ATAXIA. Unsteady, wide-based gait. Other cerebellar signs are associated.

PARKINSONISM. Stooped posture with flexed elbows and wrists. Slow, shuffling gait with short steps and stiff turns.

Facial Paralysis

	Lower Motor Neuron Lesion	*Upper Motor Neuron Lesion*
COMMON CAUSE	Bell's palsy	Cerebrovascular accident
SIDE OF FACE AFFECTED	Same side as the lesion	Side opposite the lesion
LOWER FACE	Weak or paralyzed	Weak or paralyzed
UPPER FACE, *e.g.,* raising eyebrows, closing eyes	Weak or paralyzed	Normal or slightly weak

Involuntary Movements

TREMORS. Rhythmic oscillations that may be most evident (1) on movement (intention), (2) at rest, or (3) when maintaining a posture

INTENTION TREMORS

RESTING TREMORS

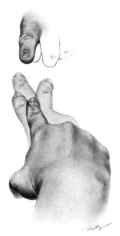

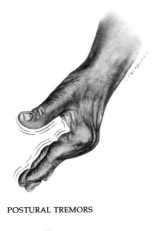

POSTURAL TREMORS

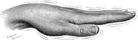

ATHETOSIS. Slow, twisting, writhing; face, distal limbs

CHOREA. Brief, rapid, irregular, jerky; face, head, arms, or hands

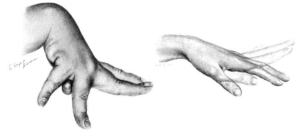

FASCICULATIONS. Fine, rapid flickering of muscle bundles

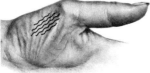

MYOCLONUS. Sudden brief, rapid jerks; limbs or trunk

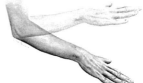

TICS. Brief, irregular, repetitive, coordinated movements, *e.g.*, winking, shrugging

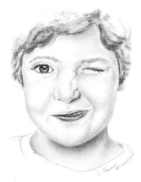

DYSTONIA. Grotesque, twisted postures, often truncal

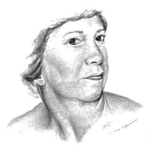

ORAL-FACIAL DYSKINESIAS. Rhythmic, repetitive, bizarre

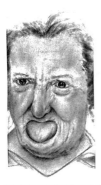

		Motor
	Lower Motor Neuron Disorders	*Upper Motor Neuron Disorders*
INVOLUNTARY MOVEMENTS	Often fasciculations	No fasciculations
MUSCLE BULK	Atrophy	Normal or mild atrophy (disuse)
MUSCLE TONE	Decreased or absent	Increased, spastic
MUSCLE STRENGTH	Decreased or lost	Decreased or lost
COORDINATION	Unimpaired though limited by weakness	Slowed and limited by weakness
REFLEXES		
DEEP TENDON	Decreased or absent	Increased
PLANTAR	Flexor or absent	Extensor
ABDOMINALS	Absent	Absent

Disorders

Parkinsonism	Cerebellar Disorders
Resting tremors	Intention tremors
Normal	Normal
Increased, rigid	Decreased
Normal or slightly decreased	Normal or slightly decreased
Good though slowed and often tremulous	Impaired
Normal	Normal or swinging
Flexor	Flexor
Normal	Normal

Dermatomes

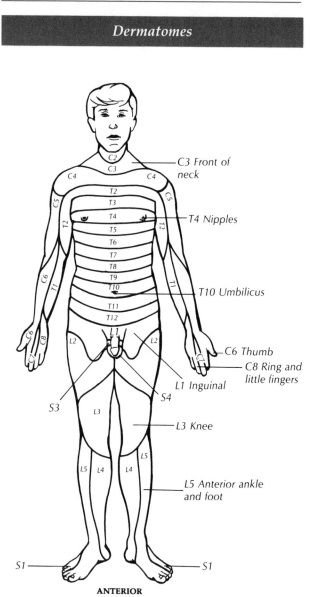

ANTERIOR

Dermatomes (Cont.)

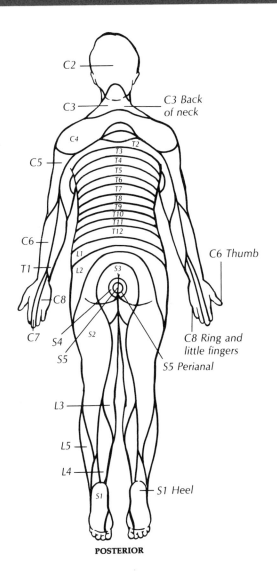

POSTERIOR

Attributes of Clinical Data

Accuracy—the closeness with which a measurement reflects the true value of an object

Precision—the reproducibility of a measurement

Sensitivity, specificity, and *predictive values* are illustrated in a 2 × 2 table, as shown below in an example of 200 people, half of whom have the disease in question. A prevalence of 50% is much higher than is usually found in a clinical situation. Because the positive predictive value increases with prevalence, its calculated value here is accordingly high.

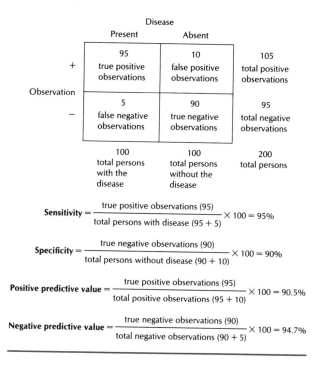

$$\text{Sensitivity} = \frac{\text{true positive observations (95)}}{\text{total persons with disease (95 + 5)}} \times 100 = 95\%$$

$$\text{Specificity} = \frac{\text{true negative observations (90)}}{\text{total persons without disease (90 + 10)}} \times 100 = 90\%$$

$$\text{Positive predictive value} = \frac{\text{true positive observations (95)}}{\text{total positive observations (95 + 10)}} \times 100 = 90.5\%$$

$$\text{Negative predictive value} = \frac{\text{true negative observations (90)}}{\text{total negative observations (90 + 5)}} \times 100 = 94.7\%$$

5

Clinical Thinking and the Patient's Record

Three parts of the patient's record are outlined in this chapter: (1) a comprehensive evaluation of an adult, from the history to the plan for the patient, (2) a problem list, and (3) a progress note. Clinical thinking is reviewed in the assessment portion of the comprehensive evaluation. Details of the history (see Chapter 1) are not repeated here. Major items in the physical examination are listed and should be expanded as indicated for a particular patient.

History

IDENTIFYING DATA, including name, address, age, place of birth, marital status, race, occupation, and religion

REFERRAL SOURCE, if any

SOURCE OF HISTORY

CHIEF COMPLAINT(S)

PRESENT ILLNESS, including

A chronological account of the symptoms and their attributes
The meaning of the illness to the patient and his or her responses to it

PAST HISTORY

General health, as the patient perceives it
Childhood illnesses
Adult illnesses

Psychiatric illnesses
Injuries
Operations
Hospitalizations

CURRENT HEALTH STATUS

Allergies
Immunizations
Screening tests
Environmental hazards
Exercise/leisure
Sleep
Diet, over a typical day
Current medications, both prescribed and over-the-
    counter
Tobacco
Alcohol/drugs

FAMILY HISTORY in diagrammatic or outline form. This should give the age and medical condition of at least the parents, siblings, spouse, and children and the age at death, with its cause, of any who have died. The family history should also include common familial or hereditary diseases and the presence of an illness similar to the patient's in any family member.

The symbols and structure of a family diagram are shown below.

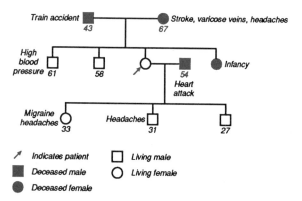

PSYCHOSOCIAL HISTORY

Home situation, significant others, and daily life
Important past experiences, such as school, work,
  marriage(s)
Outlook on the present and the future
Relevant religious beliefs

REVIEW OF SYSTEMS

General, including weight, weakness, fatigue, and fever
Skin
Head
Eyes
Ears
Nose and sinuses
Mouth and throat
Neck
Breasts
Respiratory
Cardiac
Gastrointestinal
Urinary
Genital
Musculoskeletal
Peripheral vascular
Neurologic
Hematologic
Endocrine
Psychiatric

———— *Physical Examination* ————

General survey, described in a succinct paragraph
Vital signs. Pulse rate, respiratory rate, blood pressure,
  and possibly temperature
Height and weight, in dressing gown, if possible
Skin, including skin color, texture, lesions; the hair and
  nails
Eyes. Vision, conjunctiva, sclera, pupils (size, shape,
  reactions to light), extraocular movements,
  ophthalmoscopic examination
Ears. Auricles, canals, drums, auditory acuity
Nose. Mucosa, septum, sinus tenderness

Mouth. Lips, buccal mucosa, gums, teeth, tongue, pharynx

Neck. Thyroid gland, trachea

Lymph nodes. Cervical, axillary, epitrochlear, inguinal

Thorax/lungs. Breathing (pattern, effort, sound), shape of chest, fremitus, percussion note, breath sounds, adventitious (added) sounds

Cardiovascular. Carotid pulses, jugular venous pressure, apical impulse, heart sounds, heart murmurs

Breasts. Size, symmetry, tenderness, masses, nipple discharge

Abdomen. Shape, scars. Percussion note. Tenderness, including costovertebral angle tenderness. Palpable structures, including liver, spleen, kidneys, aorta, masses

Genitalia
- Male. Penis, scrotum and contents, including testes; hernias
- Female. Vulva, vagina, cervix, uterus (size, shape, position), adnexa. Rectovaginal examination

Rectum. Anus, rectum, and (in men) prostate. Stool for occult blood

Peripheral vascular. Skin color, peripheral pulses, edema, varicose veins

Musculoskeletal. Deformities, swollen or tender joints. Back (curvatures or tenderness). Range of motion.

Neurologic
- Cranial nerves (not already described)
- Gait, tandem walking, toe- and heel-walking, hops, knee bends
- Romberg test
- Motor system (in the detail indicated): muscle bulk, muscle tone, strength, coordination, involuntary movements
- Sensory system (in the detail indicated): pain, light touch, vibration, position, discriminative senses
- Reflexes

Mental status, in the detail indicated
- Appearance and behavior
- Speech and language
- Mood
- Thought and perception
- Memory and attention
- Higher cognitive functions

——————— *Assessment* ———————

For each problem identified from the patient's history, physical examination, or laboratory studies, summarize the relevant data and outline the clinical thinking that led to your formulation. The steps in the thought processes involved in this assessment are outlined below.

- Identify and list the abnormal findings in the data base, including the symptoms, physical findings, and laboratory data.
- Cluster these findings into logical groups.
- Localize the findings anatomically as precisely as the data allow.
- Interpret the findings in terms of probable process.
- Make one or more hypotheses about the nature of the patient's problems.
- Eliminate those hypotheses that do not explain the key findings or that are incompatible with them.
- Weigh the probability of competing hypotheses according to
  Their match with the findings
  Their probability in this particular patient (of the given age, sex, habits, geographic location, and other variables)
- Consider carefully the possibility of potentially life-threatening or treatable conditions even if they are less common and thus less likely.
- Establish a working definition of the problem(s) at the highest level of certainty and explicitness that the data allow.
- Recall that various findings can be evaluated according to their accuracy, precision, sensitivity, specificity, and predictive values. Definitions of these terms are given at the end of Chapter 4.

——————— *Plan* ———————

For each problem, develop a plan in three categories:

- Diagnostic
- Therapeutic
- Educational

──────── *Problem List* ────────

This is a numbered list of problems that is usually placed in the front of the patient's chart. The name of a problem (but not its number) is modified if additional data change the assessment. See the following example.

Date problem entered	No.	Active problems	Inactive problems
9-24-90	1.	~~Edema, left leg~~	
9-25-90	1.	Deep venous thrombosis, left iliofemoral vein	
9-25-90	2.	Acute chest pain and dyspnea	

──────── *Progress Note* ────────

Include the date and perhaps the time. Give the number and name of the problem, followed by

S. (Subjective) The patient's report
O. (Objective) The clinician's observations
A. (Assessment) The clinician's interpretation of what is going on
P. (Plan) Further plans, diagnostic, therapeutic, or educational

Index

ISBN 0-397-54783-8

90000

9 780397 547838